Story of the Lotus

In Buddhism, the lotus flower is a symbol of purity, growth, and enlightenment. Its colorful petals open on long stalks that grow in muddy waters.

"The lotus flower is a magical flower, for it is rooted in mud, surrounded by water and yet somehow finds a way to bloom and grow. A lotus is a survivor. It pushes its way through muddy waters and finds the sunlight. As the bud hits the surface of the water and drinks in the sunlight, a single petal opens, signifying an achievement. Oftentimes in our busy lives, we overlook the smallest achievements. Each petal that opens is an achievement of survival, life, and opportunity. A lotus has strength and beauty. It is able to overcome all of its environmental obstacles and show the world its beauty."

Shayna Fujii *LOTUS Psychological Services*

embrace
your wobbles

Wisdom from the Yoga Mat

essays edited by
Priscilla Shumway

Editing, Design and Distribution by Bublish, Inc.

Paperback ISBN: 978-1-64704-250-9
eBook ISBN: 978-1-64704-251-6

CONTENTS

EDITOR'S PREFACE

BY PRISCILLA SHUMWAY

"May the entire universe be filled with
peace and joy, love, and light.
May the light of truth overcome all darkness.
Victory to that light."
Sri Swami Satchidananda

I HAD BEEN practicing yoga for sixteen years before I first heard the expression *Embrace your wobbles*. I had just completed writing a book—*Real Women, Real Leaders*—in which I was a co-editor and had managed a variety of contributing authors on the topic. I had enjoyed the process and found that a book written by more than one expert on a subject offers a wider lens on that subject. I believed that this format would likewise work well for *Embrace Your Wobbles*.

The purpose of this book is to help readers understand that wobbles (physical and mental challenges) are an unavoidable part of both yoga practice and life itself. The book asks readers to think about the types of wobbles they experience in life, both on and off the yoga mat. The book invites readers to consider how they view these wobbles, including the inner dialogue they use when experiencing one, since this often provides insight into how wobbles are perceived. Perceptions as to whether wobbles are good, bad, or neutral partly determines our response. Finally, this book challenges readers to become more aware of their habitual, often unconscious approach to managing wobbles both on and off the yoga mat.

The art of writing or editing a book is a practice. For some people, the physical practice of yoga is a solitary one. For me, I enjoy the comradery of a class with an understanding teacher. Like my yoga practice, the process of writing a book is one of collaboration. Working with the contributing authors on this book has brought me great joy. Their enthusiasm and encouragement have helped me to deeply understand the concept and value of wobbles in their lives and mine.

The format of this book is a series of essays in which experienced yoga teachers and practitioners provide their perspectives on wobbles, both in their yoga practice and in their lives. While each essay offers a slightly different perspective on the concept of wobbles, the common theme across all essays is that wobbles are an integral part of our lives. It is in noticing these wobbles, not judging them, that we continue to learn and grow. Thus, wobbles are not just unavoidable but are essential to growth.

Each essay brings a unique perspective to the discussion of wobbles, both on and off the mat.

◈ In *Always a Beginner,* I maintain that no matter how experienced you are on the yoga mat, bringing a beginner's mind to each yoga session allows you to be more present to the experience of the moment. On and off the mat, maintaining a beginner's mind facilitates the ability to notice but not judge the experience of the moment and to respond as needed.

◈ In the essay by Dr. Marjorie Woollacott and Dr. Anne Shumway-Cook, *Why Wobbles Matter,* they discuss how the process of learning to manage wobbles (physical and mental challenges) changes the very structure and function of the brain itself.

◈ The Rev. Dr. Elaine Peresluha's essay, *Embracing Vulnerable Patience,* suggests that the strategies learned to manage wobbles on the yoga mat (such as acceptance and surrender versus contraction and resistance) are the same strategies used when faced with wobbles off the yoga mat.

◈ In *The Spiritual Perks of Falling Apart,* Rachel Scott writes about her journey from a life which had fallen apart to her yoga practice that became a doorway through which she began to heal.

◈ A powerful dream brought Barrie Risman insight into her habit of self-criticism and her deep sense of unworthiness. She shares in her essay, *Turning Toward the Self,* how her hatha yoga practice played an essential role in shifting the nature of her inner dialogue from critical to compassionate.

- Carol Krucoff shares in *Navigating Health Challenges* how her yoga practice has helped her though multiple health issues—from a brain tumor to heart issues. As a yoga therapist, she knows firsthand the positive effects yoga has on her patients.
- In *Shaping Our Perceptions,* Richard Rosen shares his eighteen-year journey with Parkinson's Disease and how these wobbles have inspired his creativity with a wide variety of props he uses when teaching yoga classes.
- In my essay, *Balance, Memory. and Eagle Pose,* I explore the relationship between working memory and poses such as the eagle pose, which challenge balance. I propose that noticing the wobbles in balance is important to the process of improving balance and working memory.
- The effects of yogic breathing can be seen in reduced blood pressure and can change our emotional state, as explained by Dr. Sundar Balasubramanian in his essay, *In the Middle with Prana.* Pranayama is a door to accessing the deeper levels of our consciousness.
- In her essay, *It's the Mystery, Not the Mastery,* Jo-Ann Staugaard Jones explains the connection of the physical, emotional, and spiritual wellbeing that a yoga practice brings.
- Muni Natarajan, a former Hindu monk, explores what it means to be a human *be-ing* rather than a human *do-ing.* In his essay, *Centering: The Stillness*

of Balance, he describes a practice of centering which finds stillness in balance.

- ✥ For my essay on *The Path of Least Resistance,* I share my thinking of a wobble as a call to action, but there are usually multiple options for responding to any wobble. How do I decide which is appropriate for me at that moment, on that day?

- ✥ *Mountaintop Enlightenment*, an essay by Christine Wushke, uses the metaphor of climbing a mountain—both the ascent and the descent—and how nature teaches us to embrace the dark along with the light. Wobbles are as essential to us as darkness and light.

This book can be read from front to back, or you can choose to read the essays out of order. I hope this book challenges you to notice and not judge the wobbles you experience both on and off the mat. I hope you will realize that wobbles contribute to your ability to stay balanced and cultivate a sense of peace, equanimity (an inner calmness under pressure), and joy in your life.

My never-ending thanks goes out to all of the yoga teachers who have touched the lives of the beginners, those who are new, and those of us who show up on the mat daily. Thank you for helping people understand that yoga isn't just a physical practice but an entire system for living. My hope is that those students who go to "phys-ed " yoga classes come to realize that the eight limbs of yoga will not only help you *embrace your wobbles* but to also stay balanced and flexible in both your body and in the way you live your life.

Stay on the mat. Stay open to learning about this ancient system for living a moral and loving life. Stay open to the changes that will occur daily, weekly, and when least expected. Stay open to the humor and the tears on the mat. Stay curious. Stay away from judgment. Find a great teacher, one who can adjust your pose and touch your heart. One who embraces your wobbles and their own.

See you on the mat!

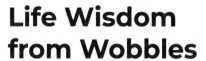

Life Wisdom from Wobbles

THE ESSAYS IN this section remind us that yoga is many things to many people. To some, yoga represents a wonderful way to exercise their body. Practice of the asanas (yoga postures) has a beneficial impact on the physical body, increasing strength and flexibility, improving balance, and enhancing stamina. But, in fact, within yogic traditions, the self has many layers— the layer of the physical body, the emotional and mental layer, the energetic or pranic layer, and a central core of pure awareness. Patanjali, an ancient Indian sage, defined eight limbs of yoga practice. He described these as a systematic way to impact each layer of the self, through which we can develop an inner state of peace, equanimity, and presence, which is experienced not only on the yoga mat but within our daily lives. Essays in this section of the book consider the different reasons that draw people to the practice of yoga and explore how the breadth of yogic practices can satisfy the many intentions bring people to the mat.

Patanjali also defines yoga as the stilling of the "fluctuations of the mind." Fluctuations impact each layer of the self, including the physical body (such as when we lose balance during a challenging pose), the mind and emotions (when our thoughts wander and our emotions fluctuate), and the prana/energy (which includes fluctuations in our energy and regulation of the breath).

These essays also explore the different types of wobbles encountered both on and off the yoga mat and discuss the importance of wobbles and the lessons we can learn when we pay attention to them. The essays suggest that wobbles are neither good nor bad but are rather an essential element in the process of growth.

Finally, collectively, these essays help us understand how lessons from the yoga mat can inspire us to seek new avenues and perceptions in life as well as in our yoga practice. Yoga may lead us on a spiritual journey in which we celebrate the accomplishment of a new pose, notice our inner dialogue when we struggle with wobbles, and learn how to accept wobbles as the first step in learning to adapt to them.

"Yoga is a practice of transforming and benefitting every aspect of life, not just the 60 minutes spent on a rubber mat; if we can learn to be kind, truthful and use our energy in a worthwhile way, we will not only benefit ourselves with our practice, but everything and everyone around us."

EMMA NEWLYN EKHART YOGA

ALWAYS A BEGINNER

BY PRISCILLA SHUMWAY

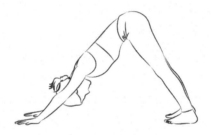

For this hour, I will honor my breath.
For this hour, I will honor my body.
For this hour, I will be grateful to my body and
my breath for bringing me onto the mat.

IT WAS 2003, and I was in my first yoga class. It was a small studio with mirrors on the front wall. I had borrowed a flimsy mat, the lights were low, and the smell of incense brought me back to the 1970's dorm room vibe. Yoga was just becoming popular in Charleston, South Carolina. A new friend had invited me to go, and we tried it out together. At the end of the class, as I lay on my mat in shavasana, I found myself in tears. How could this simple "exercise class" bring me to such an overwhelming release of emotions? What was this "Om" all about? What do you mean there are eight limbs? I have four and boy, did they ache! Thus, I began my journey into the practice and study of yoga.

Within a year, I had traveled to McGill University for a weekend intensive workshop with the world-renowned yoga teacher Donna Farhi. Sitting in the dorm room with my fellow yogis, I pestered them with questions about their journeys, what books they recommended, and what types of yoga they practiced. The class was packed with all ages, sizes, and abilities. It was a transformative weekend. I read Donna Farhi's book, *Bringing Yoga to Life,* and have returned to it repeatedly over the years. A passage I come back to repeatedly as a guiding principle in my spiritual journey is:

> *"Rediscovering who we really are at our core*
> *opens the way to experiencing our most basic*
> *level of connection with others. It is the opening*

of the heart so that we have the capacity to feel tenderness, joy, and sorrow without shutting down. It is the opening of the mind to an awareness that encompasses rather than excludes."

Fast forward to 2016. I was in an early morning class and we were doing the "tree" pose. Several students had a hard time maintaining their balance that day. The teacher encouraged us to be curious about our experience of balance during the various poses, to notice yet not judge it, and to use the wall or other props, as necessary.

"Embrace your wobbles, folks," she said. We all laughed. But with the laughter came an awareness of several valuable lessons. First, encouraging each student to notice but not judge what is happening at that moment is an incredibly important practice both on and off the yoga mat. Each moment, as we enter into a pose, we are the only person who can decide what is right for us that day, that moment. Providing options for each pose, with suggestions as to how to go deeper or to find a modification, allows students to become aware of their experience and decide for themselves which option is most appropriate—go deeper or modify. Encouraging students to honor but not judge *their* practice is crucial to the ability to respond rather than just react to the wobbles of the moment.

The second lesson was the awareness of maintaining a beginner's mind both on and off the yoga mat. According to research done by Fitts and Posner, there are three stages to skill development. When we are first learning a skill, such as practicing a new yoga pose, the beginner's mind focuses on understanding the nature of the pose and developing effective strategies in performing the pose. This stage requires a high degree of cognitive activity, such as attention, and is called the *cognitive stage of learning*. In balance poses, wobbles are inevitable. Especially in this first stage of skill development, the mind strays and muscles may easily fatigue.

The second stage continues to be very cognitively demanding and involves the refinement of strategies used to perform the skill. In this stage of yoga, we may understand the names of the poses and be able to do them without watching the teacher. We may also focus on alignment and breathwork. It is important that wobbles occurring in this stage be understood as neither good nor bad. Rather, wobbles help us pay attention and improve.

The third and final stage of skill acquisition has been called the *autonomous stage*. Performance is now much more automatic, requiring few attention resources. While doing the poses may feel more automatic, our attention may wander, so we are merely completing the postures without our full attention or intention.

When we maintain a beginner's mind, we are more likely to notice—to bring the experience of the moment into our conscious awareness. The beginner's mindset enables us to respond to the needs of the moment rather than just react automatically. No matter how experienced one is, bringing a beginner's mind to each yoga session allows you to be more present to the experience of the moment. On and off the yoga mat, maintaining a beginner's mind facilitates the ability to notice but not judge and respond as needed.

As you read these essays on wisdom from the yoga mat, absorb them with a beginner's mind. How has your experience as a yoga student or practitioner benefitted from having a beginner's mind? For we are all beginners. Each day, with every new experience both on and off the mat, we experience each moment anew.

As Donna Farhi explains, "Yoga is the startling and immediate recognition of our basic sameness. It is the practice of observing clearly, listening acutely, and skillfully responding to the moment with all the compassion we can muster. And it is a homecoming with and in the body, for it is only here that we can do all these things."

The Woollacott/Shumway-Cook essay brings a unique neuro-science perspective to our understanding of wobbles. These authors discuss how the process of learning to manage wobbles both on and off the yoga mat changes the very structure and function of the brain itself. And now for a disclaimer! Dr. Anne Shumway Cook is my sister. She and Dr. Marjorie Woollacott have written one of the most successful textbooks on balance and gait in use in physical therapy programs today.

WHY WOBBLES MATTER: SCIENTIFIC EVIDENCE AND APPLICATIONS TO YOGA

BY DR. MARJORIE WOOLLACOTT
AND DR. ANNE SHUMWAY-COOK

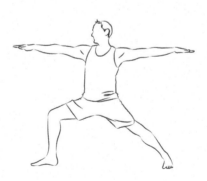

WHETHER WE ARE practicing postures on the yoga mat or carrying out the many activities required by our daily lives, we are often faced with challenges to our "balance," which we could term wobbles. In both cases, we intend to maintain balance and equanimity. Yet a variety of forces act to pull us off balance, away from our intention. To understand how to gracefully navigate these challenges to staying centered, it is helpful to explore more deeply the meaning and goal of *yoga* and the possible ways in which wobbles contribute to our ability to sustain balance.

The Sanskrit word *yoga* means *union*. It is derived from the Sanskrit root *yuj*, which means *to join* or *unite*. In the western world, we typically associate the word *yoga* with the systematic use of postures (asanas) to exercise the body, improving strength, flexibility, and balance. This focus on learning to move into and maintain asanas is typically called hatha yoga. However, the word yoga is most accurately understood to refer to a system of practices developed in India and codified by the sage Patanjali, designed to bring about peace of mind and, ultimately, union with our highest self. Patanjali defines yoga as the "stilling of the modifications of the mind," with the goal of resting or abiding in our true nature, which is pure awareness. In this system, hatha yoga is just one element, along with others such as concentration and meditation, used as tools to attain a peaceful inner state. Different people bring different intentions to the practice of yoga. Some come to the yoga mat with the intention of improving physical function (strength, flexibility, and balance). For others, the practice of yoga is one element within a broader set of practices designed to cultivate and maintain an inner state of stillness, presence, and equanimity in their daily lives.

How do wobbles contribute to our ability to achieve the intention we bring with us to the yoga mat? For many people, wobbles are considered a hindrance to achieving the goals of their yoga practice. Alternatively, wobbles could be perceived not as "good" or "bad," but rather as an element in the process of growth. Let's consider the role wobbles might play in the two different intentions. First is the intention to improve physical function such as balance. Second is the intention to cultivate and maintain a specific inner state.

When learning to maintain various poses on a physical level, a wobble may be seen as a disturbance to one's physical balance—displacement of the center point of the body beyond the base of support defined by a specific pose. These challenges to balance can be frustrating, but interestingly, research has shown that the process of developing good balance requires that we lose balance over and over again! The brain's capacity to change in response to experience is called neuroplasticity and is fundamental to our ability to adapt to challenges. Thus, the brain requires wobbles (loss of balance) to improve the neural control of balance.

Have you noticed in your practice that you spend a lot of time resisting and contracting against wobbles? Resistance is often an indicator that wobbles are perceived as harmful rather than helpful. Also, resistance to wobbles may indicate that our intention is more focused on our ego's need to attain mastery of a pose rather than to be present with equanimity to whatever is happening in our practice of yoga. For example, as you practice the tree pose *vrkshasana* while standing on one leg, you may experience both fear and frustration—fear that a loss of balance will require you to return your second leg to the mat to prevent a fall, and frustration that you have "failed" to master the pose. What if, instead of working to resist wobbles and align the posture, you noticed wobbles without judgment, remembering that wobbles are an essential part of neuroplasticity. Wobbles help the brain improve balance by giving us the awareness of the limits of stability inherent in each pose. Wobbles in themselves are neither harmful nor beneficial but instead may be considered a healthy and natural part of yoga practice. Why else would we call it practice?

What is the role of wobbles during meditation? In this case, a wobble can be seen as a movement away from the ultimate intention of yoga, which is the stillness of mind, equanimity, and presence. In our meditation practice, we find that there are two kinds of wobbles. In one case, there is too much effort. For example, there may be too much determination focusing on the breath. Too much effort may lead to rigidity of mind and a sense of contraction. In the second kind, there is too little effort, which also leads to wobbles, now related to loss of focus and attention. In either case, wobbles may induce a sense of frustration that we are not meditating "correctly." Perhaps believing we will never achieve a sense of mastery, we may quit in response to that feeling of frustration.

There is fascinating research examining the effects of meditation on the neuroplasticity of the brain, including how the brain deals with mental wobbles—the tendency of our mind to wander during meditation. The presence of mental wobbles is an integral part of a neural circuit that underlies our ability to maintain and recover a focused, centered, still point of awareness in meditation (Ricard, Lutz, and Davidson, 2014).

Using brain imaging, Davidson and his colleagues examined the moment-by-moment neural processes activated during meditation. Participants were asked to lie in a functional MRI and focus their attention on the sensation produced by breathing. Typically, during this form of meditation, the mind wanders from the breath, the object of focus. When the meditator recognized that mind wandering had occurred, he or she pressed a button and brought his or her attention back to the breath. The researchers identified four phases within a meditative cycle, each involving a specific brain network. A description of the particular neural processes affected by meditation is provided in the appendix.

The person begins meditation with a focus on the breath. When a distraction occurs, there is increased activity in what scientists call the wide-ranging default-mode network (DMN)[1] of the brain. The DMN is thought to be our normal or default mode of thinking and is responsible for the constant narrative that goes through our mind during the day. This narrative may also be considered the basis for our ego, encompassing the stories we create about ourselves and the world around us. The second phase in the process of recovering from the wobble of mind wandering is to become aware of the distraction. This involves other brain areas[2] called the salience network. The third stage occurs in additional areas[3] of the brain, which are engaged to "take back" one's attention by detaching it from any distracting stimuli. The fourth stage involves other networks[4] in the brain that help the meditator return attention back to a focus on the breath. Thus, repeated experience with mental wobbles (mind wandering) during meditation changes the neural circuitry necessary to cope with challenges to an inner state of stillness, equanimity, and presence.

Meditation not only increases resilience (the ability to return quickly to an inner state of equanimity in the face of challenges), it is associated with changes in the neural circuitry correlated with compassionate action. The practice of meditation increases a sense of unity and interconnectedness which, in turn, increases both compassion and altruism. [6] Researchers have shown that rather than becoming depressed by suffering, people who meditate are five times more likely to act to reduce suffering in others as compared to those who do not meditate. [6]

Neuroscience research suggests that the process of managing wobbles begins with awareness. This awareness includes both the actual detection of the mental wobble and an understanding of our emotional reaction to it. A wobble perceived as harmful results in the emotions of fear and frustration (usually associated with the thought, "I am not good enough and will never achieve mastery over this") and the tendency to struggle against the challenge. Alternatively, a wobble perceived as challenging but a healthy and natural part of a practice is more likely to foster an open, relaxed, and curious attitude (associated with the thought, "This challenge is a part of growth and is necessary to my practice"). This understanding is not automatic and is not always easy, but it is an important part of learning to constructively adapt to challenges.

Yoga encompasses a system of practices whose ultimate intention is to cultivate an inner state of stillness, equanimity, and presence, not just on the yoga mat but in all aspects of daily life. The wobbles we encounter both on and off the yoga mat appear to be a necessary part of this process.

The Rev. Dr. Elaine Peresluha's essay suggests that the strategies she has learned to manage wobbles on the yoga mat, such as acceptance and surrender as opposed to contraction and resistance, are the same strategies she has learned to use when faced with wobbles off the yoga mat. Rev. Elaine was the transitional minister for five months at the Unitarian Church in Charleston. We shared many hours talking about our yoga practice and its role in our lives.

EMBRACING VULNERABLE PATIENCE

BY REV. DR. ELAINE PERESLUHA

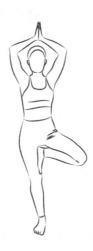

"Your life is a sacred journey. It is about change, growth, discovery, movement, transformation, continuously expanding your vision of what is possible, stretching your soul, learning to see clearly and deeply, listening to your intuition and taking courageous challenges at every step along the way. You are on the path...exactly where you are meant to be right now...and from here, you can only go forward, shaping your life story into a magnificent tale of triumph, of healing, of courage, of beauty, of wisdom, of power, of dignity and love."
Caroline Joy Adams

TWENTY-FIVE YEARS AGO, I was in a particularly challenging place—managing my midlife, being newly divorced and a single mom, all while in seminary. I was stressed by the spiritual tumult of theological education and the financial and emotional reality of single parenting. My task, as I see it now, was to let go of life as I had known it and embrace the wobble of change. I depended on running to manage my stress. One particularly beautiful fall day on Cape Cod, I was about five minutes into my run when I distinctly heard a voice.

"You do not have to keep running."

I stopped and listened while my whole body flooded with relief. Tired of avoiding pain, tired of running away, tired of rushing, I was ready to slow down, feel the reality of my life, and let my soul catch up with me. I finished that life-changing mile walking at a leisurely pace. My first lesson had been learned. Don't run. Don't resist your reality. Embrace it. Embrace the wobble.

A week later, I said *yes* to my first yoga class. I discovered it was a practice that could balance my mind, body, and spirit. My second lesson had been learned. Embracing my wobbles rather than running from them allowed me to find the time, the money, and the courage to practice something new. In yoga, I found all the elements of growth that challenged and inspired me physically, emotionally, and spiritually. For twenty-five years, I have practiced stretching myself, loving my Self, expanding the limits of my body, my mind, and my spirit. I have leaned ever more deeply into opening my heart and mind to give and to receive.

The art of hatha yoga is practiced with the eyes open, for only with our eyes open can we truly see where we are and where we want to go. That works with wobbles, as well! I have been continually amazed at the number of times I have felt as if my foot is in the proper position or that my body is straight, only to look with eyes open to discover my toes are pointed out or my leg is twisted. In a headstand, I cannot feel if I am leaning to one side. The eye of my instructor is needed to right me because I am unaware if I'm leaning to one side or the other. Intention and practicing with eyes open are required to stand straight or to stretch myself into being long before jumping my legs into any asana. Preparation is everything. With eyes open, we rightly feel the wobbles.

Before I learned this, without preparation, without intent, my eyes would automatically shut tight every time I attempted a handstand. My head would thump against the wall. For months, my teacher watched.

Gently, she would notice and say, "Open your eyes."

I wouldn't. I couldn't.

"Open your eyes. You are struggling without knowing where you are going," she said.

Bingo. She called me on my life habit—struggling without looking, without knowing where I want to go. I finally heard her. I opened my eyes. I saw the blank wall, felt my fear, stretched my body long and jumped my legs up. Up I went without bumping my head. In shutting my eyes, I had invited illusions, fear, and the control of my unconscious mind, inviting my body and my wobbles to reside outside of my awareness rather than seeing them and embracing them as part of my practice. Now, both on the mat and off the mat, I practice keeping my eyes open, locating myself intentionally in the moment.

Wobbles invite our attention and our intention. Wobbles ask to be accepted just as they are, not exaggerated or diminished.

They are part of the moment in which we reside, and only at that moment can we appreciate them, embrace them, and work with them as a tool. Wobbles teach us who we are and where to find our balance. Our minds are brilliant! They want to trick us into feeling in control when we need to let go. That is an essential lesson to take from our mats into our lives. I get to choose moment to moment how to engage with my wobble, to appreciate the lesson each wobble brings to my awareness of my Self and the world around me. My practice every morning reminds me whether or not my life is in alignment or if something is out of balance. Yoga instantly reminds me whether I am resisting or embracing my wobbles.

In tree pose, I fall over every time, unable to keep my heel on my thigh or my arms raised. Yoga has taught me that a prop—a wall or a belt—can help me to find my balance and experience the completed pose, even though I may not have the physical flexibility or strength to hold it on my own. I can build my strength and flexibility with help until I can hold the pose without a prop. Off the mat, this has taught me that it is okay to ask for help, to allow my wobble to welcome receiving support with the same feeling of competence and generosity with which I give support to others. That has always been my challenge—to feel comfortable about needing help.

In seeking alignment of the limbs and joints, we must be not only be grounded to the earth, we must also simultaneously reach upward. We stretch between possibility and all the realities which bind our bodies, minds, and spirits. Yoga embodies the dynamic tension between being rooted and stretching out beyond the limits of our awareness. It is about knowing how far to stretch without causing injury. Understanding when pain is a sign of growth and movement or when it is a sign of danger or injury. Sometimes a pose demands a stretch from the left side of the body to the right side of the body, from the rational to the intuitive. Every pose has its counterpose which demands the opposite stretch, always seeking balance in our body, mind, and spirit.

The practice of yoga has convinced me that our fundamental attitudes toward life have their physical counterparts in our bodies. I'm convinced because I see a direct relationship between my practice and my emotional wellbeing. When I stretch myself emotionally, challenge myself to go beyond my emotional, spiritual limits of honesty, appreciation, and compassion, my poses reflect the emotional effort. My poses are effortless. My joints open, and my muscles are stronger.

Yoga master B.K.S. Iyengar says, "…comparison and criticism must begin with the alignment of our left and right sides… tenacity is gained by stretching limbs in various poses for minutes at a time while calmness comes with quiet, consistent breathing…continuity and a sense of the universe come with the knowledge of the eternal presence of tension and relaxations…the eternal rhythms of inhalation and exhalation, creating a cycle of life."

Every wobble in each different asana teaches me. Inversions, handstands, headstands, shoulder stands, and forearm stands demand that I let go of fear. When our world is upside down, life demands a shift in perspective, reaching for something new, the unknown. Letting go of attachments and the familiar does not come naturally to us. It requires courage, strength, and trust. Seeing the world upside down may open us to new possibilities of peace and acceptance. For me, it allows the truth of a situation to be revealed.

We may feel the results of emotional tightness, fear, and resistance to the wobbles all around us, from global economic imbalance to the immigration crisis to environmental degradation and the Black Lives Matter movement. Contraction is what happens in our bodies and minds when we choose to avoid or power though our wobbles rather than be open and vulnerable and allow the wobble to guide us to a new level of self-awareness, integration, and balance. Sometimes our wobbles don't invite action, but instead invite vulnerable patience and an embrace. As a minister, a parent, and a partner, this is the greatest gift my wobbles have given me, both on the mat and off. Acknowledging, accepting, and living according to my wobbles has grown my ability to experience the moment, whether it offers pain, an unexpected challenge, a simple joy, or profound insight.

Wobble. Enjoy this moment. It is all we ever have.

Rachel Scott reveals a personal journey from a life that had fallen apart to her yoga practice that became a doorway through which she began to heal. She came to understand that wobbles help us to focus less on external perfection and more on our internal resources and understand that we are intrinsically worthy. In her yoga classes, she invites her students to embrace their wobbles and reframe their experience.

THE SPIRITUAL PERKS OF FALLING APART

BY RACHEL SCOTT

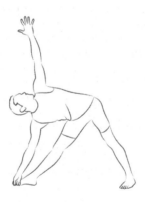

*"Out beyond ideas of wrongdoing and right
doing there is a field. I'll meet you there.
When the soul lies down in that grass, the
world is too full to talk about."*
– Rumi

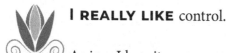 **I REALLY LIKE** control.

As in…I love it.

When the world starts to slide, my impulse is to batten down the hatches. I make lists, design spreadsheets, and straitjacket anything that feels wobbly. With steely-eyed determination, I impose order on chaos and bring entropy to its knees!

Naturally, this doesn't always turn out very well.

The biggest shakeup of my life occurred in 2006, when I left a blooming life in New York City to get married and move to Vancouver, Canada. I'd never been to Vancouver before, but my boyfriend was Canadian and wanted to return home for our future together. My leap of faith felt romantic, exciting, and inspiring. What joy it was to leap into the unknown!

However, my leap ended with a plunge into an abyss.

Just before we arrived in Canada, my husband—an alcoholic who had been dry for more than a decade—experienced a shattering loss when his mother died and started drinking again on our honeymoon.

My life suddenly got very wobbly.

Before the move, I had identified myself as an empowered and successful woman. I had a rising career in my community, a happy home, and was proud to be a New Yorker. In the space of a few months, I had moved to a new country, changed jobs, and was witnessing the unraveling of my marriage. As my husband continued to drink, I became frozen in uncertainty. I lacked the tools and resources to support his grief and became shut down in the spotlight of his anger. He mistook my silence for apathy, and our spiral of miscommunication drove the marriage to its breaking point.

All the labels to which I had been anchored (New Yorker, strong woman, kind person, and committed partner) fell apart. The external labels that had given me my sense of self dissolved. And at the same time, my weaknesses were crowbarred open and exposed. It was like pulling up the floorboards of my internal basement—a lot of dark, slimy corners were suddenly exposed to light. Who was this enabling, wimpy, silent, contracted shell of a woman? Where had the devoted partner and staunch feminist gone? I was a crab out of my shell—vulnerable, raw, weak, and exposed.

That year was also one of the best things that has ever happened to me.

When my life fell apart, I simply couldn't pretend I had it all together any longer. Nothing in my outer world was steady. No amount of list-making could bandage up the reality that I was standing in ruins.

When my outer world fell apart, my inner world started to become visible.

"The arrival of chaos should be regarded as very good news," according to Trungpa Rinpoche, the Buddhist meditation master.

When something comes along to rock our lives and challenge our sense of self, we get scared and angry. We often stuff our feelings with Netflix, potato chips, or, as Brene Brown so insightfully notes in her TED Talk, "a few beers and a banana nut muffin." When my world fell apart, I buried myself in work and started going to raves to avoid the void. Being a workaholic felt productive and validating. Dance parties and drugs were a quick fix where I could feel excited, loved, and connected.

But eventually I realized I couldn't stay high forever. When I finally sat down with my wobbles, I realized they hadn't disappeared. Even though I had separated from my husband and was no longer a New Yorker, there was something else within me that was still safe and whole. But I could only feel this steadiness—my Presence—when my control strategies fell apart.

My yoga practice became a doorway through which I began to heal. On the yoga mat, I could release the need to be in control and practice staying present moment to moment. No matter how shaky I felt, yoga invited me to be in my body—and stay there, one breath at a time. On the mat, I didn't have to be strong, happy, optimistic, perfect, or even courageous. I only had to be. My yoga practice didn't care if I had my outer life together—it only asked that I be present and feel.

For thousands of years, yoga philosophy has recognized our tendency to misidentify ourselves with the outer world. In the opening of the seminal yoga text, *The Yoga Sutra*, Patanjali explicitly lays out his definition for yoga. Here's a rough paraphrase: "Yoga is the quieting of the fluctuations of your mind. When you do this, you can experience your Presence. Otherwise, you think you're all the stuff in your head!"

Before I moved to Vancouver, my sense of Self was intrinsically tied to how I thought about myself. Was I smart? Pretty? Hardworking? A failure? Accomplished? My sense of "Rachel" was defined by my achievements and shortcomings. When those identifications fell apart, something else had the opportunity to be seen.

When we quiet our minds, our true Self—our Presence—becomes visible. But usually, we're so caught up in protecting these identities that we can't experience our depths. When our identifications get shaken, when the wobbles occur, a space cracks open where we can question our stories. You have probably experienced this during a career change, relationship shift, or a conflict. The wobbles give us the opportunity to rediscover who we are.

"Only to the extent that we expose ourselves over and over to annihilation can that which is indestructible in us be found," said Pema Chodron, Buddhist nun and author.

So, here's the good news—our lives don't have to be annihilated to reconnect to our Presence. Thank goodness! By engaging in some consciously self-imposed wobbling, we can practice reconnecting to our Presence every day. Yoga is a great place to start.

When we wobble physically on our mats, our instinct is to cover it up. The ego takes over, and we want to hide from appearing imperfect. For example, if we feel wobbly in tree pose, we may grab the wall or rigidly brace ourselves. If we fall, we look around to see if anyone saw us.

Perfect. At that moment, we can notice our attachment to getting it right or looking good. It's another time when we define our worth by something external. When our minds create stories and the ego gets flustered ("I'm a loser," or "My balance sucks!"), we should recognize that we are still intrinsically okay. In my yoga classes, I invite my students to embrace their wobbles and reframe their experiences.

I say, "If you fall out of the pose, the first thing I want you to think is, *I'm sexy! Falling is sexy. Being wobbly is sexy, because it means you're willing to go someplace that is uncertain, and that's so much more wonderful than being afraid to move out of your comfort zone!*"

The mini wobbles we experience on our mats can help create space to reconnect to a more profound identification with who we really are.

When we meditate in our yoga practice (whether it's a formal meditation or a mindfulness practice), we have the perfect opportunity to witness our minds in action. As thoughts arise, we can begin to notice they are not reality. When we see how much flotsam and jetsam is coming and going all the time across our consciousnesses, we may choose not to take what the mind tells us quite so seriously. Instead, we can begin to settle into the space that lies between our fluctuating thoughts.

When we practice questioning the mind on the mat, we have more space to question our stories *off* the mat. When our egos are threatened, there is greater grace and deeper resources to recognize that we–and those around us—are still intrinsically worthy. When life falls apart (a job loss, the end of a relationship, broken heart, or loss of a loved one), it becomes easier to pick up the pieces. Or we may even realize that we can leave the pieces where they are because we don't need them to experience who we truly are.

Embrace your wobbles. Shake your tree. And amid that wobbling, discover the unshaking ground that lies beneath and within you.

A powerful dream brought Barrie Risman insight into her habit of self-criticism and her deep sense of unworthiness. Her hatha yoga practice played an essential role in shifting the nature of her inner dialogue from critical to compassionate. How she overcame her inner wobbles is an engaging and hopeful story. Her story resonated with me, as I often find self-criticism can undermine our sense of self-worth and our power.

TURNING TOWARD THE SELF

BY BARRIE RISMAN

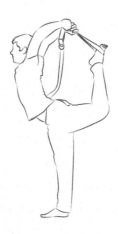

Lead me from the unreal to the real,
Lead me from darkness to light,
Lead me from death to immortality.
- Bṛhadāraṇyaka Upaniṣad

I HAD BEEN a student of meditation for several years when, in 1997, I moved to India for a long-term stay at the ashram of the path I had been practicing. A few weeks after I arrived, I was invited to offer *seva* (selfless service) as the kitchen manager, overseeing the preparation and service of all meals for hundreds of people. Since I had only recently arrived, the Indian culture and cuisine were still new to me. I didn't even know the Hindi names of the vegetables. There was so much to learn! I knew this was going to be a time of significant expansion for me.

My fellow yogis did their best to support me as I learned my new role, and, from the beginning, everything went well—at least it appeared so on the outside. All the meals were tasty and on time, and there was always enough food for everyone. But inside, my long-held habit of self-doubt was in full swing. Instead of being grateful for all the support I was receiving and appreciating the daily marvel for everything that was going *right*, I kept focusing on the mistakes I was making and how much I *didn't* know. Little did I know it at the time, but I was under the spell of months-long wobble away from my true capability, my power, and my sense of self-worth.

One day while resting after lunch, I had a powerful dream. In the dream, I was sitting across a desk from my meditation teacher. She was interviewing me, as if for a job. Somehow, I knew she was interviewing me on my ability to change. After a series of questions, she looked directly into my eyes and with great tenderness and love, I heard her say, "You are so great, but no one will ever know it unless you change."

In the weeks and months following my dream, I spent time inquiring into the inner turmoil I was creating. I realized something crucial. At the root of my habit of self-criticism was a deep sense of unworthiness. I felt that no matter what I did, no matter how smoothly the kitchen ran, I would never be *good enough*. As a result, I could never be happy with myself as I was. I discovered that a lack of self-worth was at the core of my feelings of frustration, failure, and incapability.

I had heard the teachings that said, in effect, "You are great. You are whole. You are perfect just as you are." Intellectually, I knew they were the truth. But did I believe it deep down inside? I realized that even more than giving myself a break from the constant voice of self-criticism, I needed to change how I saw myself as an individual. I had to change my relationship with myself. To step into my greatness, I had to let go of the thoughts, habits, and tendencies that kept me limited, unworthy, and small.

These, of course, are all ways we tend to wobble away from what yoga tells us is our true nature, the greatness, wholeness, and perfection that lives in the heart of every human being. From that moment on, nurturing and building a loving relationship with myself became a significant theme in my *sadhana,* my spiritual life.

My hatha yoga practice played an essential role in shifting the nature of my inner dialogue from critical to compassionate. Asana became a practice of self-honoring and self-acceptance. I used it to cultivate a loving relationship with myself. I consciously related to my body as an instrument for the inner work of yoga and ultimately as the vehicle for service to the highest. Over time, I started to experience my body as strong and beautiful. I recognized it as sacred, worthy of love and respect, a temple for the divine. Taking care of my body felt like an offering. Postural practice became an expression of self-love and respect.

This is an example of the power of approaching yoga as a practice of nurturing a loving inner relationship. I believe that yoga practice is at its most transformational when we use it as a way to restore, nurture, and expand a loving, compassionate relationship with ourselves. We do this not only for ourselves but also because doing so changes the way we see others and interact with the world around us.

At some point, even the most assiduous yogis are likely to wobble away from feeling worthy and whole in one way or another. The good news is that experiencing these kinds of inner wobbles can open up new avenues of inner examination. They may inspire our longing for empowerment, growth, and self-discovery. Deep-seated feelings that somehow, we just aren't good enough just as we are, are often at the root of our search for something more. They can compel us to dig deeper and seek out ways to nurture self-acceptance, bringing about feelings of wholeness.

In my experience, wobbling away from our inherent worthiness can show up wearing many disguises, including:

- ✦ Persistent self-criticism
- ✦ A habit of comparing oneself with others, usually coming out on the bottom end
- ✦ Feeling discouraged, disempowered, defeated, and hopeless
- ✦ A lack of self-confidence
- ✦ Taking things personally
- ✦ A feeling of underlying sadness, even when everything seems to be going okay
- ✦ Loneliness, even amidst others

Yoga offers us an alternative way of relating to ourselves and our wobbles, one that is grounded in a vision of the human being as inherently complete and whole. Through practice, we gain glimpses of this state that, over time, fortify our conviction that, indeed, we are good enough.

We do this not only by thinking and feeling that we are good enough but by actually embodying this idea. Through intention, movement, and breath, we install the vision of ourselves as supremely worthy of receiving love into the fabric of our bodies. We become capable of listening to and dismissing the nagging inner voice that tells us we'll never be good enough, knowing full well it is not the real story.

We learn to embrace our wobbles with the tenderness of a mother holding her child. In these ways, we nurture a compassionate, loving relationship with ourselves that is bigger than what our mind tells us. At the same time, we strengthen the recognition of our essential worthiness by taking hold of the teachings that tell us we are—and always have been—perfect exactly as we are. We let go of the need for outer approval and recognize our inherent goodness.

Noticing Your Inner Wobbles

In the years that followed my dream and the subsequent period of transformation I experienced, I thought about the dynamics at work in yoga that supported me in creating lasting and authentic inner growth.

The space of our practice offers two ways to work with our wobbles that together create the possibility for a shift:

⬧ *Welcoming what is:* Yoga practice gives us a place to meet, see, feel, and thoroughly be with reality (both internal and external) *as it is*, without pushing it away, judging it, or wishing it could be different. Just being with it. This includes bodily sensations as well as the full range of the mind and emotions—the usual mental chatter of moods, thoughts, and reactions and stronger emotions like anger or fear.

✧ *Going beyond what is:* At the same time, practice gives us access to an inner space that is slightly apart from the reality of what is. This is the space of witnessing. It is the firmament, the all-encompassing awareness that holds the fullness of our experience and yet is not affected by it, like the sky is unaffected by clouds. Shifting to this awareness provides us with the critical perspective needed to feel our independence from what is happening. This space of witness consciousness is the self-reflective capacity that exists within every human being and is the beginning of yoga's path to inner freedom.

In anthropology, this is called being a *participant-observer.* An anthropologist immerses himself or herself in a culture while at the same time remaining separate enough to observe that culture. Similarly, yoga teaches us how to be aware of what we are thinking and feeling while at the same time knowing we are more than just what our minds tell us.

As in the months following my dream, the practice of working with our inner wobbles in this way and coming back again and again to our innate strength and worthiness fosters conviction. It empowers us to face life's challenges with resilience and steadfastness.

Integrating Wobbles into Your Practice

Another crucial element of facing our wobbles and turning toward our true Selves is having ways to integrate our experience of yoga practice into the rest of our lives. Integration is about digesting and assimilating what we experience in yoga. It's about letting the lessons of our practice seep into our consciousness and then bringing them into our way of living in the world, weaving them into the fabric of our everyday lives.

The truth is that everything about the way we approach yoga is a metaphor for life. When I'm patient with myself on my mat, it's easier for me to be patient with my daughter. When I'm accepting of myself in yoga, it's easier for me to accept others as they are. When I feel nurtured by my practice, it feels natural to nurture my family and others. When I'm able to dance with my wobbles on the mat, I get better at responding to them in my life.

Integration happens when we approach all parts of our lives—including family, relationships, work, the way we process current events or how we rake the leaves in our backyard—through the lens of our experience and understanding of yoga. We learn to approach every moment, every situation, as an opportunity for practice. Coordinating our breath rhythm with our steps while taking a walk, softening our shoulders and relaxing our posture to feel more at ease while sitting in traffic, or remembering the farmers who grew our food while preparing a meal to enhance our experience of interconnection—these are all examples of infusing yoga into the rest of our lives. We bring consciousness, breath, awareness, and a recognition of a larger, grander, and even sacred purpose to every encounter, to all our tasks and situations. Over time, there is less and less separation between our yogic selves and who we are in the rest of our lives.

Adapted from *Evolving Your Yoga: Ten Principles for Enlightened Practice,* by Barrie Risman, 2019

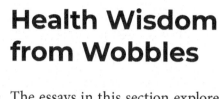

Health Wisdom from Wobbles

The essays in this section explore how yoga can benefit us as we face health challenges. The health benefits of a yoga practice that includes postures, breathwork, and meditation are many. Previous and ongoing research has shown that yoga can help with mental and emotional health, improve balance, establish better sleep patterns, and reduce stress. The American College of Physicians has recommended yoga as an option for chronic low back pain and other medical and psychological conditions. In fact, yoga is now classified by the National Institutes of Health as a recognized and accepted form of Complementary and Alternative Medicine.

These essays explore ways in which adapting various yoga practices have helped practitioners to manage health wobbles. Examples of helpful adaptations include using props when balance is compromised or meditating before surgery to calm the mind and body. Essays also explore the effect of different aspects of yoga on the physical body (improved balance, reduced blood pressure) and the mind (improved working memory).

The essays also discuss the process of managing health wobbles, with awareness as the first step. It is through awareness and attention to our emotional reactions to health wobbles that we learn to adapt and manage them. Do we struggle against these challenges or do we acknowledge them, exploring how to adapt to them both on and off the yoga mat? By learning to accept and adapt to health challenges, we cultivate the ability to maintain stillness, acceptance, and gratitude in all conditions.

Finally, these essays explore the effects of health challenges on both our yoga practice and, more broadly, on our lives. They also consider how a yoga practice can help us adapt mentally, physically, and spiritually to health challenges. As Nischala Joy Devi, yoga teacher and healer, says, "What you say, feel, think, and imagine, makes a huge impact on the outcome."

Acknowledging the wobbles in our bodies and finding alternative ways to practice poses helped two of the authors create new routines in response to health challenges. Cultivating a sense of gratitude and ease in the body and mind can influence our internal environment and reduce suffering. Accepting help, whether it be from other people in our lives or the use of props on the mat, may help us to find equanimity and steadiness when faced with the challenges of life.

In sharing her story of experiencing various health wobbles, Carol Krucoff explains how the practice of yoga helped her to navigate and thrive. She describes how her yoga practice offered profound teachings, since a central focus is finding equilibrium — that steady place between effort and surrender. Living with medical issues can be a powerful daily practice. As a yoga therapist and instructor at Duke Integrative Medicine, Carol teaches and counsels from personal experience.

NAVIGATING HEALTH CHALLENGES
BY CAROL KRUCOFF

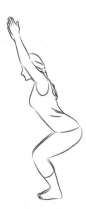

"Health is wealth. Peace of mind is happiness. Yoga shows the way."
- V. Saraswati

THERE'S NOTHING LIKE facing a heart procedure to help you forget about your brain tumor—and vice versa. Like many people in our aging society, I find myself—at age sixty-five—with a surprisingly long "problem list" on my medical chart, including:

- A prosthetic heart valve, which I've had since 2008, when I underwent open heart surgery to replace my congenitally abnormal aortic valve and to repair a resulting aneurysm.

- A benign brain tumor called an acoustic neuroma on the nerve responsible for hearing and balance. Discovered as an incidental finding in 2003, it slowly grew over the years and has been stable since 2014 when I had Gamma Knife radiosurgery.

- A history of atrial fibrillation, an abnormal heart rhythm I lived with for several years before having two cardiac ablations that restored normal rhythm—for the moment.

Despite these scary-sounding conditions, I am blessed to have excellent health insurance and medical care, to be very fit and, in general, to feel great. I walk my dog several miles and practice yoga every morning, teach yoga classes, and take ballroom dance lessons. Several of my physicians have speculated that my healthy lifestyle may have contributed to my doing so well with my varied medical challenges. Yoga has proved extremely helpful in navigating these health wobbles—those distressing periods where my body reminds me that it won't last forever.

USING YOGA TO PREPARE FOR SURGERY AND ENHANCE HEALING

As a yoga therapist at Duke Integrative Medicine in Durham, North Carolina, I'd often helped clients deal with the stress of difficult health conditions through relaxation breathing, meditation, and appropriate yoga postures. So, before my heart surgery in 2008, I designed a practice to help ready myself physically, emotionally, and spiritually for the challenges, drawing upon Patanjali's Yoga Sutra II:33, which states, "*When presented with disquieting thoughts or feelings, cultivate an opposite elevated attitude.*"

In the six weeks I had to prepare for my surgery, my daily routine included *pranayama* (three-part breath and extended exhalation), deep relaxation, and meditation on a positive outcome. My asana practice changed according to my needs— some days, it was dynamic and energizing, other days calming and restorative. During meditation, I imagined myself going through the procedure successfully and then visualized myself celebrating my birthday the month after the surgery, healing and happy and surrounded by family and friends. I often prayed, asking for help and strength to bear whatever was to come.

I loaded up my iPod with guided meditations and my favorite Sanskrit chants. I listened to these during my preoperative cardiac catheterization, while being wheeled into surgery and in the Intensive Care Unit (ICU). Becoming absorbed in the chants helped calm my fears and find strength in connection with my unchanging True Self.

Three months after my surgery, I was back to teaching yoga, and today I am grateful to feel fine. Surgery is one of life's major wobbles and can also be a profound opportunity for growth. Mine offered many lessons, including a renewed appreciation for the precious gift of breath. Facing mortality drives home the reality that our time on earth is limited and has inspired me to declutter my home and my life—making conscious choices about how I use this finite resource. In my morning meditation, I have added to my three *oms* two *moos* to honor my prosthetic bovine (cow) heart valve. And, perhaps most important, is the renewed recognition that yoga is about much more than asana (postures). My experience taught me that even when you can't move—lying in an ICU bed, for example—you can still practice yoga. Breathing, meditating, and chanting can all be powerful healing practices.

WATCHING MY LITTLE BRAIN TUMOR GROW

I learned about my acoustic neuroma brain tumor by accident in 2003 around my fiftieth birthday. Fortunately, my tumor was a benign and generally slow-growing type. The specialist

I consulted recommended two possible treatments—brain surgery to remove it or radiation to stop its growth. But since I had no symptoms and the tumor was tiny, I chose a third option—*watch and wait*, which meant having annual MRIs but avoiding treatment unless symptoms appeared or progressed. *Watch and wait* doesn't mean doing nothing, because routine surveillance involves wobbles—some physical, some emotional, and some financial. And it requires a tolerance for uncertainty, the willingness to live with something that could either be a ticking time bomb or a harmless growth.

In navigating the wobble of living with a brain tumor, again I turned to my yoga practice to help me remain relatively calm over the years as I watched my tumor's creeping growth—at the rate of about 1mm (the size of a grain of sugar) each year. Walking an emotional tightrope between responsible vigilance and anxious obsession, I gratefully clung to the fact that I had no symptoms—my hearing and balance appeared unaffected. Yoga offered profound teachings since a central focus is finding equilibrium—that steady place between effort and surrender. This is also the key to watchful waiting—doing whatever is possible while accepting that not everything is possible. Also, regular practice of balance postures may have contributed to my balance remaining unaffected, even though tests showed that the vestibular function in my affected side was abnormal. Fortunately, there is a paired nerve on the other side of the brain which my doctor said might have taken over for the damaged nerve as I continued to practice balance poses daily.

At my annual MRI in 2014, I learned that my tumor measured about 1.2 cm, about the size of a small walnut. Continued growth could mean a strong likelihood of adverse effects on my hearing and facial nerves. I decided to have a type of radiation therapy called Gamma Knife radiosurgery. My yoga practice helped me get through the morning-long outpatient procedure. Relaxation, breathing, and mental chanting helped me lie very still in the Gamma Knife Unit, which was similar to having an MRI. By the following week, I felt fine and was back to teaching yoga. I'm grateful to have had no adverse effects from the procedure, and annual MRIs have shown that my tumor is stable.

Like me, more people in our aging society are "incidentally" learning about hidden abnormalities. While us humans have always been aware of our mortality, we have never been able to so clearly see the train that may take us out coming down the track. For me, this unsettling knowledge presents a spiritual opportunity. Like the ancient yogis who were taught to imagine Death sitting on their shoulders, having a heightened awareness of impermanence may serve to make the present moment that much sweeter. Rather than being morbid, the recognition that life is fleeting can be a joyful daily practice of gratitude, celebrating the precious gift of breath.

ADVENTURES IN A FIB

One day in 2011, my regular heart rhythm changed to chaos—an irregularity called atrial fibrillation, or AFib. While AFib itself is usually not life-threatening, it dramatically increases the risk of stroke if left untreated and may lead to other problems, including heart failure and chronic fatigue. My heart surgery put me at increased risk, as did my age. While some people with AFib don't know they have it, others—like me—are acutely aware when their heart rhythm shifts from steady to disorganized. Feeling your heart thump wildly in your chest can be frightening, exhausting, and sometimes disabling.

In some ways, my experience with AFib was the ultimate "circular" health wobble, because stress can trigger AFib and being in AFib causes stress. This makes it extremely important to address the emotional aspects of living with the condition, which I did through my yoga practice and by consulting a therapist.

I developed strategies which allowed me to do almost everything I needed to do regardless of my heart's rhythm. I rarely canceled an appointment or class because I was in AFib. I taught yoga and gave presentations with a chair nearby so I could sit if my racing heart made me lightheaded or too tired to stand. Then, in 2014, after a lengthy episode where my heart did not revert to normal rhythm on its own, I was hospitalized for a cardioversion, a procedure where electrical currents shock the heart back into a normal rhythm. I was ready to try a more invasive solution that might provide more lasting relief, deciding to have a cardiac ablation in January

2015. The procedure restored my normal rhythm for about eight months, when I again woke up in AFib. I had a second ablation several months later and, thankfully, have been in normal rhythm since.

HONORING HEALTH WOBBLES

Living with health wobbles can be a challenging daily practice involving gratitude for the gift of breath and having faith that, even if a condition can't be cured, healing is still possible. And I've learned that, just because you're a patient, you don't have to be helpless. Even in that most vulnerable position— wearing a flimsy, ill-fitting hospital gown—you can still influence your internal environment and reduce suffering. Breathing, meditation, prayer, and gentle movement can all help cultivate ease in body and mind.

The harsh reality is that health wobbles are an inevitable part of being human. One of the Buddha's Five Remembrances is this:

I am of the nature to have ill health. There is no way to escape ill health.

Yoga centers on this recognition of impermanence. The inescapable reality of human existence is that everything changes—except, according to many wisdom traditions, the immortal soul.

Over more than four decades of rolling out my yoga mat, my practice has undergone many changes. While I still do postures, breathing, and meditation to strengthen my body, my health wobbles have made me more attuned to the yogic teaching that our bodies are vehicles for the spirit. Now, a central focus of my practice is becoming more connected with awareness itself. In the words of the great spiritual teacher, Sri Nisargadatta Maharaj: *"You are not the body. You are the immensity and infinity of consciousness."*

When I begin to wobble, abiding in this truth helps me find steadiness and ease.

In this poignant and thought-provoking essay, Richard Rosen compares the "Chandler Wobble," the unbalanced spinning of our Earth, with the physical and spiritual wobbles we experience in our lives. Sharing his journey into yoga and his onset of Parkinson's Disease (PD) allows us to see how he has fully embraced the wobbles in his life, both on and off the mat. The health wobbles of PD have encouraged him to be more conscious of himself. His creative use of props has made him a better teacher when working with students who also have limitations.

SHAPING OUR PERCEPTIONS

BY RICHARD ROSEN

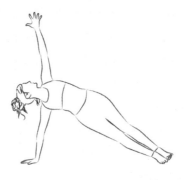

*"The practice of yoga brings us face-to-face
with the extraordinary complexity
of our own being."*
-Sri Aurobindo

BACK IN 1891, after nearly thirty years of research, an American astronomer named Seth Carlo Chandler confirmed what Isaac Newton had predicted about two hundred years earlier—that there's a "slight displacement" in Earth's rotation. What does that mean? It means our planet doesn't spin exactly straight around its axis. There seems to be some disagreement among scientists regarding the displacement's main contributing factors, though it's generally accepted that Earth's shape plays some part.

We imagine Earth is a perfect sphere like a baseball, but like all rapidly rotating celestial bodies, including stars, the North and South poles are flattened by the force of that rotation. In other words, Earth would make a terrible baseball because it's not a perfect sphere. Its diameter at the equator is about 30 miles greater than its diameter at the poles. We're all living on what's called an oblate spheroid, and, like an unbalanced spinning top, as Newton anticipated and Chandler proved, the Earth wobbles.

It's no surprise the "slight displacement" is now called the Chandler Wobble.

Now before we move on to yoga, we should look into the word *wobble* itself. I searched through at least a dozen dictionaries and discovered that wobbling has a bad rep. It's a sure sign that something's irregular, staggering, clumsy, trembling, and vacillating, not to mention all the "un-like" things it is—such as unbalanced, unsteady, uncertain, and uneven. I didn't unearth even a single kind word about wobble, not even a hint it could be useful or fun.

Yoga Sutra has a good definition of wobbling. Yoga Sutra's claim to fame is that it's the first ever presentation of a complete yoga system, usually called either Classical or Raja Yoga. It was compiled sometime in the fourth or fifth century CE by a mysterious figure tradition named Patanjali. One dictionary definition for wobble is *fluctuate*. Wobble is a word at the heart of Patanjali's teaching about yoga, which he defines as the "restriction of the fluctuations of consciousness," or, to paraphrase, we practice yoga to "stop all our wobblings."

Without going into detail, Patanjali sees wobbling as an inherent quality of material nature, which isn't just trees and dogs and rocks. He believes our consciousness (citta) is also a material process, composed of the same stuff as all that other stuff. Only citta stuff is subtler. How does it work? When our eyes fixate on a chair, for example, our citta wobbles to match the shape of the chair and other qualities, and we say, "Oh, that's a chair." But it's not our citta that ultimately makes that determination. It just thinks it does, since its "graspy" ego is always standing by on alert to pull everything into its orbit. Be that as it may, like all matter, our citta is entirely nescient. Put another way—human consciousness isn't conscious.

The way it works is that citta and its sensors—ears, eyes, tongue, etc.—receive information from both outside and inside worlds (perceptions from the former; thoughts, feelings, and memories from the latter) and pass both along to our True Self, the actual knower. Since it has no substance, our Self never wobbles, but ironically, unless it has some connection to something that does wobble, it has nothing to know and nothing to know with. This is what the English mystic-poet William Blake meant when he said (and I paraphrase), "I see *through* my eyes, not with them."

The problem is that the wobbling is much more alluring than the static Self, and we're irresistibly drawn to it like a moth to a flame—and you know how that usually turns out. This misconception, treating the wobbling self as if it were the True Self, leaves us with a powerful but inexplicable feeling of loss and so burdens our life with an unremitting existential sorrow. Patanjali's solution, then, is the only one that's feasible—to end the sorrow and be ourselves as we truly are by severing our association with wobbling nature, which includes our body.

Patanjali's solution takes the form of the well-known eight-limb (ashta anga) practice. After some preliminary work to drain away as much of his emotion as possible, the experienced practitioner trains himself, with the help of the guru, to sit stock still for hours on end, barely breathing or not breathing at all (inhales and exhales are perceived as wobbles). With his senses withdrawn from the outside world and redirected inward to his citta, he now seals himself in a self-created cocoon. Nothing gets in and nothing out.

Inside the cocoon, he gradually learns to focus all his attention on a single point, the wobble of which grows subtler and subtler over time until one glorious day the last wobble drops away. He then emerges from his cocoon, not as a beautiful, fluttery butterfly—that world to him no longer exists—but as an immaterial, quality-less nomad, bound to remain in blissful, self-absorbed, un-wobbling isolation for eternity. (Just to be clear, the views expressed in this part of the story are not the author's but are entirely those of Patanjali and his commentators.)

As an Iyengar-trained teacher/practitioner, I spent my yoga babyhood studying the Yoga Sutra, which is the Iyengar school's traditional guidebook. Since that school places a heavy emphasis on asana performance, I learned very early on in my teacher training that, according to Patanjali, not to mention Mr. Iyengar, wobbling in yoga was everything the dictionaries said it was—and that went double in an asana. For an Iyengar student's asana, nothing less than *steady and comfortable* was acceptable, and even then, there was always some question. After all, *today's maximum is tomorrow's minimum.*

So, I pushed myself and was driven by my teachers to *strengthen that back leg*, or *reach up through the heels*, or *firm the outer arms inward.* The wobbling slowly diminished as I felt I was rounding myself not so much toward fulfilling the concept of *steady and comfortable*, as I had no illusions about my overall ability in asana, but at least toward a bearable level of wobbliness.

Then in 2002, after twenty-two years of practice, the wobbles returned in a brand-new shape, grinning madly, and this time they were here to stay. The first sign something was changing was a constant numbness in my toes. Next came the occasional shuffling gait and the bouts with depression. I was diagnosed with Parkinson's Disease (PD). PD makes you weaker, stiffer, and wobbly. After all the thousands of hours I'd spent getting myself strong, flexible, and evenly keeled, I came to the conclusion that the universe has a very wry sense of humor.

My practice changed considerably (as did my life), and with it my understanding of wobbling. Slowly but surely, the wobbles crept back into my practice and my life. I had two choices—I could punch and counterpunch with every steady and comfortable anti-wobbly boxing move I'd learned over the years, or I could try something radically new and just accept them.

I was sure the wobbles didn't have my best interests in mind, but I could see the futility in trying to knock them out. I reluctantly welcomed the new wobbles as being as natural to me as they are to Earth (and now, at age seventy-two, my belly, like Earth's diameter, is growing more oblate every day).

It appears that after eighteen years, the strategy is working fairly well. There's no doubt the condition is advancing, but at a rate my PD doctor deems "ridiculously, miraculously slow." He always insists it's "your yoga" we have to thank, but I'm not so sure. It could be that, or my new leaf approach, or maybe I'm just plain lucky. On the bright side, the wobbling has inspired my creativity with a wide variety of supportive props, blocks, straps, chairs, sandbags, wedges, blankets—you know, everything a yoga teacher needs to change a light bulb. It's supplied me with extra tools to help other celestial bodies— my students—with similar conditions. Maybe someday I'll come up with a word not exactly extolling wobbles but at least something that gives them some credit for being of some use under some limited conditions.

But I also must admit the wobbling has encouraged me to be more conscious of myself. I've found that a Patanjali-like focus on the wobbles when they're acting up serves to calm them down, and I don't even need a cocoon. They've also made me more aware of my surroundings, shuffling down a city street with full PD is akin to navigating an especially devious obstacle course. Cracks, tree roots, and curbs are hiding everywhere to trip me up. Not being a perfect sphere, then, is a mixed bag, but I always remember what my favorite yogi, Yogi Berra, once wisely opined: "If the world was perfect, it wouldn't be."

I have always been interested in understanding the physical and mental impacts of yoga and its effects on the brain. As a corporate trainer for over twenty-five years, I specialized in how the brain processes information and how we learn. Finding the correlation between improved balance and improved working memory as we age inspired this essay.

BALANCE, MEMORY, AND EAGLE POSE

BY PRISCILLA SHUMWAY

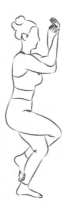

"The success of yoga does not lie in the ability to perform postures but in how it positively changes the way we live our life and our relationships."
- Rodney Yee

IT IS INEVITABLE that as we age, we will wobble more and, at the same time, be more aware of the fact that we no longer have the strength, flexibility, or resiliency of our youth. But as Mary Stewart so aptly states in her book, *Yoga Over 50,* "The aging process cannot be halted, but we do have the choice whether to conserve our health and make the most of our potential or fritter away our energies. Yoga is about the first of these choices." By practicing yoga, we are paying attention to our health—physical, spiritual, emotional, and mental. Yoga helps us to maintain our flexibility, strength, and resiliency.

Yoga helps to release tension and stiffness, and to provide balance and flexibility in the spine. By maintaining and improving our balance as we age (think fewer wobbles), we can increase our working memory. While we often choose yoga as a way to increase our balance, it may be surprising to learn that it may also improve cognitive function. In a 2017 research study by Zettel-Watson, it was found that better balance and aerobic endurance led to enhanced processing speed and working memory in older adults.

What is *working memory* and why should we care as we age? Working memory temporarily stores information that is relevant to any task we are currently doing. Wondering where you put your car keys? What was on that grocery list you left at home on the kitchen counter? This is what working memory does for us. It is the immediate skill that allows us to remember and use relevant information while in the middle of an activity. These wobbles of the working memory may be decreased by improving our balance in our yoga practice on the mat.

A 2018 article from bioRxiv stated that, "Working memory has a severely limited capacity. Humans can maintain only three to four objects at once." In other words, although one can hold anything in the mind, one can only hold a few of them at a time. Also, as balance declines with age, more of our working memory becomes devoted to balance control, specifically attending to where our body is in space so we don't fall. We rely on our attention to our balance and position in space to keep us safe, thus limiting the capacity of our working memory.

As we practice postures that stress the balance system, balance improves, thus freeing working memory for other important issues. One common source of falls as we age is trying to do two things at once. We can maintain our balance, or we can talk to a friend on the phone, but it is harder to do both without risking a fall. Knowing where our body is in space frees up working memory to pay attention to other daily tasks or where the closest Starbucks is for that cappuccino you promised yourself after yoga class (or even remembering we promised ourselves that cappuccino!).

One of my favorite balance poses is standing eagle pose. *Yoga Journal* maintains that "you need strength flexibility, endurance, and unwavering concentration for eagle pose." By practicing eagle pose, I place great demands on my balance system and work toward improving my balance both on and off the mat. I find that I physically wobble in eagle pose if my concentration and focus wobbles. Sometimes, in a balance pose, the use of an external support or a prop is helpful—and this can be a good thing!

As with many balance poses, I find I am better with my right foot as the stabilizing foot. As I wobble more on my left, I notice what my inner voice says. "Aha! Here I go again! It is so curious that my right is more stable than my left. Maybe if I concentrate harder on my focal point, or drishti, I will settle down. Perhaps I need to strengthen my core more."

But then I consider *not* trying so hard and using a block to support my right foot, therefore finding better balance. "Aha. I can use a prop today. Let go a bit, pull back, don't work so hard and get the same result. Yup, that worked. I like this pose!" I say to myself. Using a block gives me unwavering concentration. It may also help to create a new neural pathway for muscle memory. Think of the use of props on the mat like training wheels on a bike. From day to day, from pose to pose, the use of props helps us to maintain our balance with less effort, thus freeing up working memory. We can maintain our balance and enjoy the fullness and benefit of the pose. We can breathe deeper and pay attention to what is happening in the pose. Sometimes working less is more.

So, too, off the mat, understanding when support is needed and asking for it or accepting it when it is offered may be helpful. Admitting we need external support in our lives may be seen as a personal weakness or a wobble rather than a strength in life. When we are supported in friendships, at work, in our families, or in love—we may be more open to showing our vulnerabilities and sharing our truths. Asking for support, similar to admitting a prop is useful today, can be the hardest part.

And so, if we wobble less in a pose and therefore improve our balance off the mat, do we free up working memory? If we use props in yoga, can we wobble less and free up working memory? If we use props and can hold a pose longer, do we free up cognitive space to focus on our breathing, noticing our inner dialog about the pose? If we ask for and are given support in life, do we allow ourselves to feel more secure? Can we allow yoga, in the words of Rodney Yee, to "…positively change the way we live our life and our relationships?"

I'm not sure, but I am enjoying using blocks, straps, and bolsters, just as I appreciate the love and support of my beloved, my family, my yoga teachers, and my friends. I am still learning to ask for help, but just like yoga, it is a practice!

Now, how about that cappuccino you promised yourself after practice?

As explained by Dr. Sundar Balasubramanian, the effects of yogic breathing can be seen in reduced blood pressure and improved emotional status. Pranayama is a door to accessing the deeper levels of our consciousness. Along with the health benefits of yogic breathing, it helps to balance the mind. Here Sundar helps to explain how mind control can be achieved through an unwavering breath. It is no wonder that the word "prana" means breath as well as life. The breath is our life force. How yogic breathing techniques can become healing mechanisms is Sundar's life work.

IN THE MIDDLE WITH PRANA

BY DR. SUNDAR BALASUBRAMANIAN

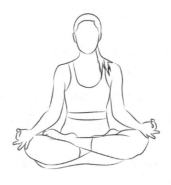

"When you do yoga – the deep breathing, the stretching, the movements that release muscle tension, the relaxed focus on being present in your body – you initiate a process that turns the fight or flight system off and the relaxation response on. That has a dramatic effect on the body. The heartbeat slows, respiration decreases, blood pressure decreases. The body seizes this chance to turn on the healing mechanisms."
-Richard Faulds (Shobhan)

When I was a child growing up in India, I had a bicycle tire. It was a dysfunctional one from my father's bicycle. It could not hold any more air due to several punctures made by roadside thorns. When he purchased a new tire, he brought the old one home for me. For most of the kids back then, owning a bicycle tire like this one was a norm. We would roll the tire on the sandy streets and use a little stick to tap it, direct it, and run after it. When the tire drifted right or left, we used the stick to re-center it to the path. The stick could make the tire roll faster with gentle taps or could function as a brake to slow it down. That was my favorite evening hobby in my childhood. The taps and brakes we applied to the tire with the stick on the left and right was the act of balancing.

Balancing a tire is like balancing the wobbles of our mind. Pranayama (the regulation of the breath through practice and techniques) is a way of balancing a wobbling mind. In fact, the wobbles of the mind can be perceived as the wobbles of our breath that goes on and off between the left and right nostrils when breathing. Our breath alternates between the left and right nostrils, and this motion reflects in the state of our mind, too. The breathing through those two nostrils is oscillating, but when the oscillation is controlled, it can bring an ultimate balance.

Of all the balances one can achieve in life, the balancing of the mind is the pinnacle. Thirukkural, an ancient text written by a secular Saint Thiruvalluvar in Tamil says, "The stature of a person who is unwavering and contented is a lot bigger than that of a mountain." An unwavering mind can achieve great heights.

Like the many highways which lead to a town, each of us has our favorite pathway on which we choose to travel. People also have their favorite ways of controlling the mind. Not everyone will necessarily work the same or work at all. The things that have worked for me in the past were being highly active, constantly surrounded by good company, and in an upbeat environment. Devotion (bhakti) and engaging in healthy habits or exercises are some other ways of controlling the mind that works for many. The mind which is not controlled has several places to wander. A wandering mind is a wobbling mind. Like a lost child, the mind is a vulnerable target. Restraining may be a strong word, but it is a powerful tool for beginners. Once the mind is tamed, we may be able to open the doors of the deeper levels of our consciousness.

Of all the methods of mind control, saints like Thirumoolar, Patanjali, several other Sithars (saints who learned the truth of life and helped people with their knowledge), and Buddha opted for breath control as a vital tool. One can easily be mindful about something close to them that is easily sensed and controlled, that goes on within the body and can be sensed instantaneously and continuously. Therefore, balancing the breath is a way of balancing the mind, as well. It allows gentle oscillation and movement, but at the same time, it keeps the mind steady with fewer wobbles and forward-looking.

MIND CONTROL CAN BE ACHIEVED BY UNWAVERING BREATH

The act of balancing ourselves has to start from the breath because that is the basis of our existence. The breath is the basis for the livelihood of the body. Alternate nostril breathing is the balance between the left and right nostrils. It is often referred to as the sun and the moon or the cold and warmth. The two contrasting natures are represented as the two nostrils. That duality of the nostrils manifests in the opposing characteristics of the physical and emotional systems of the body.

While there are no modern biological studies published or research on the concept of breathing where there is no left or right dominance (Suzhumunai), there are some studies on ida (the left nostril) and pingala (the right nostril) naadis, summarized below:

- Forcing the breathing through one nostril versus the other changes the systolic blood pressure. For instance, left nostril breathing has been shown to reduce blood pressure.

- Breathing through the nose not only supplies oxygen to the body, but also informs the brain about the smell, temperature, moisture, and speed of the breathing, and chemical contents of the air. These details are essential for the brain to react according to the environment. The nostrils may transmit opposing information to the brain. However, contrasting emotional dominance is anecdotal with left and right nostril breathing and not completely understood. But the concept of changing the emotional status with breath could be an important area for future biobehavioral studies.

- The alternation of the left and right nostrils happens once in about every two to four hours (referred to as the nasal cycle), and helps to maintain the normal physiological condition.

- Balanced, non-dominant breathing—the activation of Suzhumunai—can be achieved through the continuous practice of different types of Pranayama focusing on the nostrils' awareness.

Suzhumunai is a steady state of breath. It is the state of unwavering stability of the mind, the character with which we want to enrich our minds. Pranayama is a door to accessing the mind. It is the key to opening the doors of the deeper levels of our consciousness. Several Pranayama exercises may be a key to open this door through the realization of Suzhumunai. Alternate nostril breathing exercises demonstrate this.

1. Start by closing your eyes, then close the right nostril, slowly breathing in through the left nostril.
2. Once you complete the full inhalation, close the left nostril, open the right nostril, and start breathing out.
3. At complete exhalation, start breathing in through the right nostril.
4. When the inhalation is complete, close the right nostril, open the left nostril, and breathe out through the left nostril.
5. Repeat steps 1 through 4. You can do this exercise for ten to twenty-five minutes.

You may already know this exercise. But the key thing is that next time you do it, watch the for the following:

◈ Watch for nostril dominance—which nostril is more open than the other one? Realize there is a nasal cycle performing in the system, whether or not we are aware of it.
◈ Become aware of the breathing movement at every instance and spot, especially within your upper respiratory tract—the paranasal sinuses.
◈ Watch the movement of your eyeballs. You will be gazing at the side of the nostril that is actively inhaling

or exhaling. You don't have to purposefully try it, but you will notice it happens that way naturally.

❖ Through closed eyes, look into the middle of the forehead and sense the movement of your breathing there in the middle.

❖ Watch for any twitching at the scalp or at the tip of your ear lobes, or any other sensation, as you alternate the sides of your face as you switch nostrils.

❖ Be on the lookout for any other sensations within your entire body and mind.

Realizing the existence of duality in the physical and emotional body and sensing it through the practice of alternate nostril breathing, attaining new neutrality and, at that balanced state, keeping the mind tuned into our whole existence is the path to a fulfilled life. Like a child who runs after the bicycle tire, adjusting its speed and direction with a stick, one can use Pranayama to regulate the breath. When the breath rides smoothly like that bicycle tire, the balanced mind (like the child) will explore new pathways and noble things along the way.

> Wisdom is to none but the balanced
> Misery is not for disengaged
> Neutral ones are the divine
> I follow those that are unwavered
> - Thirumanthiram 320

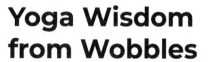

Yoga Wisdom from Wobbles

This group of essays celebrates the wisdom each person gains from his or her individual yoga journey. Regardless of our level of experience as a student of yoga, it takes us on a journey of inner discovery. On this inner journey, yoga practice is viewed as a metaphor for life. We see that the wobbles encountered on the yoga mat provide insight into how to manage the wobbles we face off the mat. We learn to apply the wisdom gained on the yoga mat to our daily lives.

These essays describe the many physical aspects involved in yoga, including the act of entering into a pose, establishing proper alignment, making the transition to the next pose, controlling the breath, and centering, all of which are important aspects of a yoga practice. They suggest that by paying attention to how wobbles affect all aspects of our yoga practice, both physical and mental, we can learn to notice but not judge these challenges and even embrace our wobbles as a lesson for growth.

The essays suggest that learning to pay attention to our wobbles on the yoga mat improves our ability to pay attention to how we respond to wobbles in our daily lives. We begin to recognize habitual patterns of behavior—thoughts and emotions that occur in response to wobbles—and explore new ways to adapt. The process of learning to adapt to wobbles both on and off the yoga mat enables us to move forward in life with gratitude. This is truly living your yoga practice. Learning to live your yoga practice means applying the wisdom and lessons learned on the yoga mat into our homes, workplaces, and communities.

As one of our authors, Barrie Risman says, "Strictly speaking, physical postures alone are just exercise. It's the context and understanding with which we perform the postures that makes them yoga."

Jo Ann Staugaard-Jones explains the connection of the physical, emotional and spiritual wellbeing that a yoga practice brings. My husband's childhood friend, Jo Ann has traveled nationally and internationally teaching yoga and yoga anatomy. She believes that yoga is so much more than the physical education version we often see in today's yoga studios. Rather, yoga connects us to our deeper selves.

IT'S THE MYSTERY, NOT THE MASTERY

BY JO ANN STAUGAARD-JONES

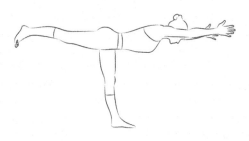

"Through sustained focus and meditation on our patterns, habits, and conditioning, we gain knowledge and understanding of our past and how we can change the patterns that aren't serving us to live more freely and fully."
– Yoga Sutra III.18

THIS is YOGA: The union, balance, and mystery of many factors coming together to quiet the roaming tendencies of the mind. (Patanjali, Sutra 1:2; the Sutras are the living source of yogic wisdom handed down through the ages.) You may have thought it was just physical exercise, but it is so much more!

In *The Secret of the Yoga Sutra,* Pandit Rajmani Tigunait, spiritual leader of the Himalayan Institute, discusses the Sutras as being as fresh today as they were 2,200 years ago, that every human being is an island of excellence, and nothing is beyond our reach. That is the Divine mystery.

As a yoga teacher and author, and for the sake of the general population of students I instruct, I like to connect yoga practices by putting them into three *compartments* (notice I said *connect*, not divide). It is the connection of physical, emotional, and spiritual wellbeing that is important.

PHYSICAL YOGA

As a graduate in Movement Sciences and a Professor of Kinesiology, I enjoy teaching Yoga Anatomy in all my workshops and classes. Still, I would be remiss if I stopped there. For many people, it is the physical practice that is most beneficial, because our society tends to think this is important. There is a real obsession with how we look, and some yogic practices capitalize on that.

In America, we also tend to be competitive and aggressive. This is when the wobbles set in. We try too hard. Our muscles begin to grip in our efforts to achieve—what? The perfect posture? There isn't one—not for *anyone*! Instead of trying to be something you're not, discover the intricacies in each asana that can help with alignment, breathing, and balance for yourself, not others. We are not robots (yet!). So, embrace your wobbles and learn from them. Notice how each asana may differ from day to day. Be aware and curious about your alignment and your breath in each posture.

Asanas are taught in classes that supposedly make us feel better, and they do! But freeing ourselves from the bonds of intensity allows us to experiment and discover much more. Remember, these postures are simply part of the journey to quiet the mind and journey inward. The wobbles of the mind and the poses are all part of the journey inward.

The deep core muscles of our body are what help us to maintain our balance. They are physically the key to embracing our wobbles! Engaging these core muscles will help steady any standing or one-legged posture (so will props!). Once steady, begin to discover the energetic quality and *mystery* of the body by being aware.

EMOTIONAL YOGA

Our emotions have developed over millions of years of evolution. They are the human response to nature, and in some ways keep us from danger. An emotional response is harbored in the brain and nervous system and is linked with survival. Brain science and a guide to the nervous system are complicated. I will focus on two techniques that calm the wobbles of the mind, muscles and nerves.

In yogic philosophy, the Yamas (restraints, or how you should behave toward others) and Niyamas (observances on how to conduct yourself) are the first two of the eight limbs of yoga, as described in the Yoga Sutras of Pantajali. From the Yamas, I believe Ahimsa and Satya are excellent starting points to begin to embrace wobbles:

- ⬧ AHIMSA = Do no harm. Have compassion for yourself and others.
- ⬧ SATYA = Truth. Understand your body and its limitations and accept them.
- ⬧ Do *not* push, pull, grip, squeeze, or tuck when practicing yoga poses. This may cause harm to your body. By understanding your body's limitations, its wobbles, in this moment, you show compassion to yourself.
- ⬧ *Do* soften, imagine, connect, change, relax, search, receive, share, create, open, extend, nourish, expand, experiment, wonder, invite, engage, spread, deepen,

transform, play, love, allow lift, balance, release, choose, grow, give, guide, adapt, surrender, and breathe!

◈ Be grateful. Express gratitude.

SPIRITUAL YOGA

It has finally been scientifically proven that there are two different levels of physical reality: the one with which we are familiar (using the five senses) and a second one termed *psychoenergetic* science. This is a level of physical reality that can be significantly influenced by human intention.

By cultivating awareness and intention in our yoga practice both on and off the mat, we begin to tap into the driving force of our spiritual practice. By being aware of ourselves on the mat—how we think, perceive, and perhaps judge our wobbles—we can use our conscious power to affect how we live our lives and interact with others. Our intention can influence our physical reality.

According to David Surrenda, CEO of Kripalu Center for Yoga and Health, "The original context of yoga was spiritual development practices to train the body and mind to self-observe and become aware of its own nature. The purposes of yoga were to cultivate discernment, awareness, self-regulation, and higher consciousness within the individual…that through compassionate self-awareness, it is possible to have a yoga practice that goes beyond the physical."

Are we on the cusp of a new scientific worldview that encompasses the growth of consciousness? We know we have many unrealized capabilities. Wouldn't it be wonderful to be able to affect reality toward a common good using a conscious power? It appears this can be addressed spiritually, mainly through yoga/meditation, metaphysical practices, and energy healing.

Muni Natarajan, a former Hindu monk, explores what it means to be a human "be-ing" rather than a human "do-ing." He describes a practice of centering that finds stillness in balance. Muni was one of my yoga teachers who made me aware of the profound effects of pranayama, chanting and meditation. His life as a Hindu monk for thirty-eight years in Hawaii and his mesmerizing drumming brings a new layer of knowledge to his practice.

CENTERING: THE STILLNESS OF BALANCE

BY MUNI NATARAJAN

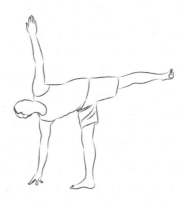

"GO FROM A HUMAN BEING DOING
YOGA TO A HUMAN BEING YOGA."
- Baron Baptiste

TO MAKE PROGRESS on the spiritual path, *being* and *doing* must come into balance with each other. If we wobble in either, we may find ourselves out of balance. While this is neither good nor bad, it is crucial to begin to notice when this occurs. Once this balance has been reestablished, there is a sense of centeredness.

When we are *not* experiencing centeredness, our awareness of *doing* overshadows our awareness of *being*. When we *are* experiencing centeredness, we are equally aware of *being* and *doing*. This concept of *doing* refers to the busyness of our lives. This concept of *being* refers to the awareness and mindfulness of our lives. When we cultivate this centeredness as an intentional practice, *being* gradually overshadows *doing* because centeredness favors *being*.

Being overshadowing *doing* doesn't mean that *doing* does not get done. It only means that *doing* gets done effortlessly from within *being* as if nothing is happening. Under the influence of *being*, *doing* occurs with maximum ease and efficiency. A valuable goal in meditation is to notice but not judge when we are *doing* rather than *being*. When *doing* becomes effortless, we know we are under the influence of *being*.

There is a beautiful yogic practice called *centering* which goes directly to the heart of centeredness. In this practice, we discover that when the body becomes balanced, thoughts and emotions also find equilibrium. This is when a three-point stabilization of body, mind, and emotion is sustained long enough to be consciously enjoyed and a calm and blissful sense of centeredness arises of its own accord. On the mat, we work toward this centering in all our poses. Off the mat, the practice of noticing our equilibrium may be interrupted by our busyness of *doing*.

The advantage of getting good at purposefully tuning into the various qualities of *being* (bliss, love, stillness, balance, peace, power, rapture, awareness, and more) is that sooner or later, we will need all of these qualities. Not all at once, of course, but separately—as the circumstances of life require. Depending on where we are in the stress and strain and wobbles of everyday living, one of these qualities will always be of more assistance to us than the others. Each circumstance of life will signal a need for a different quality until at some point in our application of yoga in life, all of the qualities of *being* will have been needed and applied so often that these qualities will have become habitual.

When yoga practices—physical, mental, or otherwise—are repeated enough to become habits, their benefits increase exponentially. As yoga habits are fed by even more repeated practice, their effects continue to grow in the domain of our unconscious life until they eventually touch the entirety of our existence. This shift culminates in what amounts to a full transformation of our nature, right down to its core.

Practices worth repeating for the habitual enjoyment of *centering* could include any well-founded yogic exercises such as pranayama, meditation, asanas, or the deeper study of the Eight Limbs of Yoga, aimed at directly experiencing any of *being's* qualities.

CENTERING PRACTICE

When we are centering, we seek to find stillness in balance. As an example, try these two physical postures called vrkshasana and sukhasana in Sanskrit.

❖ Since vrksha means tree and asana means posture, vrkshasana is often referred to in English as, not surprisingly, the *tree posture*. As you seek balance in this position, does your breath want to stop? Don't judge. Let it. Once you have become centered and feel comfortable, you can gently apply the soothing ujjayi (victorious or warrior) breath control.

Also, in this practice, we can focus on developing a seated position for meditation—sukhasana in Sanskrit. Although sukhasana literally means *joy pose*, it is usually referred to in English as the *easy pose*.

❖ Perform vrkshasana until you have established a strong sense of physical balance. Be sure to assume both the left vrkshasana (balancing on the left leg) and the right vrkshasana (balancing on the right leg).

Is your balance better on one side than the other? Do you wobble more on the left or the right? Were you more balanced yesterday? Again, don't judge it. Just notice and be curious.

- ◈ When you are finished, walk around a little bit. As you walk, try to maintain that balanced feeling you established in vrkshasana.

- ◈ After a few minutes of this balanced walking, sit down in sukhasana. In this seated posture for meditation, focus on establishing the same balance you achieved in the *tree posture* (vrkshasana). Feel how this balancing of the physical body brings calm to thought and emotion.

- ◈ Once you are comfortable and balanced in sukhasana, perform several rounds of three-part breathing (filling the belly, diaphragm, and lungs). Then relax in an ujjayi breath control as your breathing shallows.

As this natural stilling of breath is cultivated, it will encourage a further calming and balancing of mind, body, and emotion. When you sink and settle into the center of this stilling, you will experience for yourself just how fluidly and easily the yoking of yoga—the balance of *being* and *doing*—can occur. Notice any wobbles. Be curious and being aware. Discover how this yoking wants to happen and needs from you only your attention.

The wobbles of life are blessings in disguise. They usually occur when our *being* and *doing* are out of balance. They give us the perfect opportunity to return to center.

As a wise teacher from the East once said: "Stress makes you strong. In this strength, there is peace, calm, stillness, and bliss of *being. Doing* is not *being*, but it takes a lot of *doing* to be."

One of the advantages of growing older is the wisdom of hindsight. Looking back over my past, I have begun to see patterns of behavior. These same patterns play out on my yoga mat. Taking the time to notice and not judge them has brought me great insight. As you read this essay, are there patterns of behavior in your life you can identify and begin to change? Do they manifest themselves both on and off the mat?

THE PATH OF LEAST RESISTANCE

BY PRISCILLA SHUMWAY

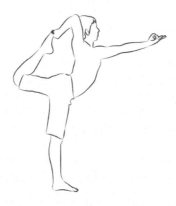

"Yoga is not a work-out, it is a work-in. And this is the point of spiritual practice; to make us teachable; to open up our hearts and focus our awareness so that we can know what we already know and be who we already are."
-Rolf Gates

I HAVE BEEN attending mostly gentle yoga classes now for a year or so—lots of easy flow, rarely a down dog, and a focus on how the breath infuses the movements. In these classes, we are encouraged to "make it your personal practice." There are always multiple options given in case a pose doesn't feel right for us at that moment. At the age of sixty-eight and having practiced yoga for over eighteen years, I find these classes fulfill my need for flexibility, mindfulness, and balance. Also, they encourage me to discern when to push hard or alternatively relax into the flow, depending on what I need in that particular moment on that particular day. My creaky shoulders and elbows love these classes.

Recently, I took a flow class for all levels which was a full-on Hatha vinyasa class with multiple down dogs and a faster pace. Looking around the class, I noticed I was one of the oldest students. I kept up with every vinyasa and sweated along with the rest of the class. As I was in the middle of the fifth down dog, I wondered how my shoulders would hold up the next day. During this class, I felt the wobbles both in my body as physical challenges and in my mind as mental uncertainty.

As I faced each challenging pose, I became aware of an ongoing inner dialogue of multiple voices, each offering an opinion on how I should proceed. Here is what I heard:

"Hey, take it easy. You don't have to prove anything. This is your practice. Take a break in child's pose."

"Oh, no. No breaks. Keep up the hard work. If you keep up these classes, you will build strength and not have these pesky shoulders and elbow problems."

"Hey, slow down. Don't hurt yourself. Is it your ego that is pushing you? Are you trying to keep up with the younger students to prove a point?"

"No, no! You always take easy classes. You know you have to build bone mass and muscle as you get older. These harder classes are good for you. The more down dogs and planks you do, the stronger you will get, and your shoulder problems will go away."

"If I hurt myself I won't want to come to class. I don't have to work so hard. I can get just as much out of the gentle classes."

All of us have multiple voices inside us. They are part of the ongoing narrative of the mind. Each voice expresses a specific opinion regarding how we should respond to a wobble (the challenge at the moment). Sylvia Boorstein, a teacher in the Buddhist tradition, suggests we name these voices. She refers to that first voice in my ongoing dialogue as the *grandmother's voice*, the voice suggesting, "Take it easy. Don't push. In fact, why not sit down and have a cup of tea!" Wisdom is understanding in every moment which voice to listen to and which to ignore. My inner dialog often vacillates between taking the path of least resistance (my grandmother's voice) versus the path that embraces the challenge. The issue of trying to discern which voice to listen to at any given moment is the lesson here.

How many voices do you hear when you experience a wobble? Which voice do you listen to, and which do you ignore?

I think of a wobble as a call to action, but there are usually multiple options for responding to any wobble. How do I decide which is appropriate for me at that moment, on that day?

FROM THOUGHT TO ACTION: DISCERNING WHICH PATH TO TAKE

In yoga, as in life, we are often faced with deciding which path or action to take from among several options that may vary in their degree of challenge. For example, which yoga class to take (easy versus hard) or the decision to use (or not use) external support during a challenging pose.

According to Wikipedia, in physics, the path of least resistance is defined as the "physical pathway that provides the least resistance to forward motion by a given object or entity, among a set of alternative paths." The path of least resistance represents the easiest course of action. It is the action requiring the least effort and resulting in the least upheaval, unpleasantness, or drama. According to numerous psychologists, humans are hardwired to take the easy route. More often, we choose to rely on experience and continue with what has worked for us before or what is most pleasant and less painful. Perhaps my love of gentle yoga classes reflects this hardwired impulse to take the easy route. While taking the path of least resistance may be our default inclination, it is crucial in life, both on and off the mat, to pause and consider if this is the right path.

In my life, I have often chosen the path of least resistance. For example, in undergraduate work, I chose to study aboard, transfer to three colleges, change my major three times, and graduate in three-and-a-half years from a very liberal college that provided me extra credit for traveling in Europe. My Master's degree was also in a new and very experimental program, with the only challenging class being educational statistics. I have not had an actual math, history, or science class since high school! I loved being a student and have been a lifelong learner. But I have not always chosen rigorous or challenging courses.

I now see that taking the path of least resistance influenced how I parented. As I look back on how we raised our two sons, I was always the one who agreed that they could quit a team sport at the end of the season rather than insisting that they stick to it. My husband felt that they needed to play organized sports to learn teamwork and that they needed to stick to a sport and persevere. I would often give in and help them write their school reports rather than nag them to finish or let them fail if they did not fulfill the requirement.

Choosing the path of least resistance may determine how we deal with a friend with whom we disagree. By not challenging them and stating our truth to avoid unpleasantness, we may be taking the path of least resistance. Staying quiet instead of confronting an issue may be taking the path of least resistance. But it is only by facing our inner resistance, ignoring our grandmother's voice, and engaging in a challenge that we grow and move forward. Wobbles exist more often on the path of greatest resistance.

"When you are challenged, you are asked to become more than you were. That means creating new perspectives, acquiring new skills, and pushing boundaries. In other words, you have to expand your understanding to be able to overcome the obstacles facing you." (Thomas Oppong, author and columnist.)

And so, on the mat and off, when faced with life's challenges and wobbles, it is vital that we pause and ask ourselves, *which path should I take*? Is this a time to take the path of least resistance or accept the more challenging path? Or is there a Middle Way?

TAKING THE MIDDLE WAY

Buddha describes the Middle Way as the path of moderation, the way between the extremes of self-indulgence and self-denial. Is there a Middle Way beyond the path of least resistance and the path of the most resistance? When faced with wobbles both on and off the yoga mat, can I find a Middle Way, neither avoiding all nor accepting all challenges? I believe I can.

Here are my Middle Way intentions:

- ◈ To notice but not judge wobbles—being aware of what is difficult or challenging in the present moment.
- ◈ When encountering a wobble (either physical or mental), to notice the inclination to take the path of least resistance and to pause and consider alternative paths.
- ◈ To challenge myself both on and off the yoga mat to engage in the challenge, not always taking the path of least resistance.
- ◈ On my yoga mat, I will practice a few down dogs and planks in every gentle class to build my strength and endurance. In more challenging classes, I will allow

myself not to complete all the vinyasas if my body tells me to rest.

⬦ To be grateful to my body for allowing me to experience wobbles, for they remind me I am still showing up to practice.

To experience wobbles in life both on and off the yoga mat is to realize we are still learning, still growing—and this is extremely important. Each day, each breath brings with it another opportunity to experience the gifts and wobbles of life!

In using the metaphor of climbing a mountain, both the ascent and descent, Christine Wushke shows how nature teaches us to embrace the dark along with the light. Like darkness and light, wobbles are also important teachers. Embracing fear heightens the senses. It instills a feeling of alertness, aliveness and heightened attention to the present moment. It is not enough to attain enlightenment, but we must try to integrate that back into our lives off the mat.

INTEGRATING MOUNTAINTOP ENLIGHTENMENT INTO DAILY LIFE

BY CHRISTINE WUSHKE

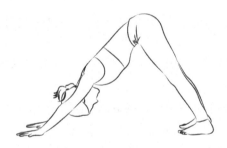

"In this very breath that we take now lies the secret that all great teachers try to tell us…the present moment. The purpose of meditation practice is not enlightenment. It is to pay attention even at unextraordinary times, to be of the present, nothing-but-the-present, to bear this mindfulness of now into each event of ordinary life."
— Peter Matthiessen, The Snow Leopard

MASTERING YOGA, SIMILAR to the development of a spiritual practice, is often compared to a journey up a mountain. So often in this metaphor, the story ends at the top of the mountain, as if, when we reach that final peak, it's *The End*, credits roll, and we all live happily ever after. As if, somehow, we can freeze time on this beautiful peak and stay in that euphoria forever. The teachings so often skipped over in spirituality are of the descent back *down* the mountain.

It's not realistic to maintain a rigid focus on reaching the goal of the mountain peak and not accept the reality that we have to get back *down* the mountain and return to the routines of our daily life. In yoga, this metaphor represents how the quest to attain enlightenment as a high state of bliss and perfection often misses the important aspect of the integration of that state back into our daily lives and everyday moments. The value of embracing wobbles both on and off the mat is that it can teach us how to more fully accept our humanity, including our mistakes and our shadows. This allows us to bring the gifts attained in yoga to these darker aspects of our humanity. In this way, we realize a state of wholeness and fullness, accepting the totality of our human experience instead of trying to cut away the dark shadows and only accept the light. When approaching yoga in this more integrated way, all wobbles have value. Learning to love our wobbles can make the journey more enjoyable. And it ultimately leads to a more complete experience of yoga as we integrate its gifts back into our lives and learn to embrace the wobbles off the mat, as well.

Any mountaineer will tell you that as much joy as there is in standing on that summit, what goes up must come back down, and a descent, while hard, brings with it its own joys. Because the sun is often setting during the descent, it may illuminate the mountains in a truly magical way. You'll get to see and feel the raw, real fullness of the mountain. Its slopes and edges are emphasized in the evening's deep shadows. It is in these moments that nature teaches us to appreciate and embrace the dark along with the light. For many people, both darkness and descent bring with them fear. But in this situation, it is necessary to befriend fear and take it with us into the adventure. Avoiding fear on these stretches of the mountain may make a hiker more vulnerable to the dangers, as avoidance of this authentic human experience limits our ability to be fully present to the experience of the moment.

What I have learned in the mountains is that fear actually heightens the senses. It instills a feeling of alertness, aliveness, and heightened sensation to the present moment. When we avoid noticing fear and other types of wobbles in our lives, we lose a valuable lesson that our body and mind are sending us. For example, when fear is embraced rather than avoided, the gift of fear (heightened sensation and alertness) comes along with it. Embracing our wobbles opens them like a gift we have unwrapped so we may receive the inherent value they have to offer us. Heightened learning, humility, self-acceptance, and a larger capacity for self-love become increasingly available the more we embrace our successes along with our failures.

These days, I'm a bit more interested in the *mountain descent* kind of enlightenment—the kind of enlightenment that doesn't exclude anything. The kind that takes the high and bright experiences from the mountaintop and brings them back down into the shadowy nooks of the forests and valleys encountered on the descent. Deep insight and wisdom are available to those who are willing to stay 'til dark and bravely listen.

The peaks are indeed euphoric. Standing there gazing across the vast expanse of the world is exhilarating and inspiring. The quality of awe and beauty is one I find difficult to express in words. But to me, the best part of the journey is the descent, where the authentic wildness of nature demands the dismantling of our innate arrogance. When looked at from this point of view, even wobbles—the negative aspects of our experience—when embraced without judgment offer us a special gift...as if a reward for including them on the journey. Wobbles such as fear, exhaustion, and weariness offer the gifts of presence, humility, and surrender. As on the yoga mat, wobbles teach us to pay attention, be curious, and enjoy the moment. The ability to surrender in a pose and be present to our breath offers us a special gift.

In summary, enlightenment isn't an endpoint. It isn't a summit to reach. If the mountains have taught me anything, it is that there is an unrelenting presence available in every moment, not just on the mountain top—a presence that gives us the endless capacity to feel the depth of all emotions—not just the pleasant ones. This presence is there in each breath, ready to carry us into and through both the highest joy and the deepest pain. And, maybe most importantly, it is this presence that allows us to find the smallest, darkest, scariest places and to love them all the way home. These are the moments to which we can all connect and relate. They bind us together and keep us united in our shared humanity. Don't try to stay there on that peak, disconnected from your humanity. Come back down and reach for the hand of a loved one. Share in the tragic beauty of what it is to be human. Embrace the wobbles which connect us all.

Appendix

Author Bios

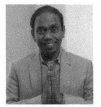

Dr. Sundar Balasubramanian is a Cell Biology researcher currently studying cellular and molecular mechanisms involved in resistance to cancer therapy at the Medical University of South Carolina. He is also a Yoga Biology researcher and is the Founder and Director of PranaScience Institute. Sundar's yoga research has provided scientific evidence on how yoga breathing practices may promote wellbeing in health and disease. His first book is *PranaScience: Decoding Yoga Breathing*, and his latest book is *Mind Your Breathing: The Yogi's Handbook with 37 Pranayama Exercises*. He also recently produced an audio album, *Chanting Is Pranayama*.

He was a speaker at TEDx Charleston 2015, and his video is among the most popular in the field (666,000+ views). This JC Bose Memorial Awardee's work is well-publicized through *Discover* magazine, *The New York Times*, *Huffington Post*, *National Public Radio,* and other popular media. His website is *PranaScience.com*, and his books and audio are widely available online, including at *Amazon.com*.

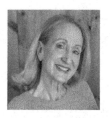

Carol Krucoff, C-IAYT, E-RYT, is a yoga therapist at Duke Integrative Medicine in Durham, North Carolina, where she offers private sessions, workshops, and classes for people with health challenges. An award-winning journalist, Carol served as founding editor of *The Washington Post's* Health Section and her articles have appeared in numerous national publications, including *The New York Times, Yoga Journal,* and *Reader's Digest.* She is the author of several books, including *Yoga Sparks:108 Easy Practices for Stress Relief in a Minute or Less* and *Healing Yoga for Neck and Shoulder Pain.*

She is codirector, along with Kimberly Carson, of the *Yoga for Seniors Professional Trainings* designed to help yoga teachers work safely and effectively with older adults. She and Kimberly are co-authors of the book (and DVD), *Relax into Yoga for Seniors: A Six Week Program for Strength, Balance, Flexibility and Pain Relief.* Along with Kimberly and Jim Carson, she is coauthor of *Relax into Yoga for Chronic Pain: A Mindful Yoga Workbook for Finding Relief and Resilience.*

She has served as a consultant on several yoga research studies and coauthored articles in peer-reviewed medical journals. Carol studied martial arts for ten years and earned a second-degree black belt and the honored title Sensei. She has practiced yoga for more than forty years and is grateful to have studied with numerous master teachers from around the world. For more information, visit www.healingmoves.com.

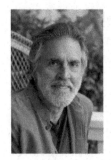

Muni Natarajan is an artist, writer, teacher, and musician. His work is deeply influenced from his thirty-seven years of practicing yoga and meditation as a monk in a monastery on the island of Kauai, Hawaii. The primary focus of his monastic life was a deep study of the Vedic origins of Hinduism as well as an ancient and traditional practice of yoga, deeply rooted in the time-honored traditions of India's ancient Vedic past.

During his monastic years, Muni served as a primary teacher of younger monks. He conducted workshops for seekers visiting the monastery and was a teacher and guide on the monastery's travel/study programs to India and other global destinations. Muni also worked as a graphic designer and editor for *Hinduism Today* magazine, and studied the Indian musical system of *ragam* and *talam* while learning tabla and mridangam drumming and classical Indian singing.

Muni departed the monastery in 2007 to marry his wife, Mary Beth. During the launch of this new life, Muni self-published two books, *A Monk's Tale* and *Into the I of All*, and composed the music for his first album, *Trance in Dance*. He then started a yoga and meditation school in Charleston, South Carolina, where he taught until 2019.

Today, Muni lives in Yellow Springs, Ohio with Mary Beth and his dog, Cody. He is currently working on a new series of Ganesha paintings and plans to launch a full schedule of meditation workshops in 2020. His ultimate intention is to do as his guru did—help students find inner peace and contentment amidst everyday challenges while seeking self-realization in the practice of Raja yoga. His website is: https://yogawithmuni.com

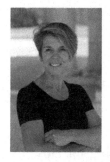

Rev. Dr. Elaine Beth Peresluha resides in Denver, Colorado. She has been an ordained Unitarian Universalist minister for over twenty years. Yoga is the daily spiritual practice which inspires her life and work. For over twenty-five years, yoga has increased her personal and professional ability to be effective, joyful, and balanced. For eight years, Elaine served in settled ministry and then chose interim ministry as a professional specialty. As in interim, she completed her PhD in Social Science, focusing on the use of Appreciative Inquiry as an effective organizational change tool. She was accredited as an interim minister in 2010 and began *In the Middle Consulting* in 2013 to expand her work with other organizations in transition. Elaine is a qualified administrator for the *Intercultural Development Instrument,* which increases the intersectional skills of congregations centering marginalized identities. In her work to support congregations and organizations through transitions, she helps to increase their diversity and inclusivity with intercultural skills.

If you are an Enneagram person, Elaine is a quintessential 7. If you prefer Myer-Briggs, Elaine is an *INFP*. A skier, hiker, and biker, where fresh air tends to her spirit, Elaine also spends time every day inside on her yoga mat. You will find her to be a warm, energetic, collaborative presence.

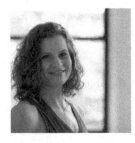

Barrie Risman is widely regarded as one of Canada's most highly-skilled yoga educators, teacher-trainers, and mentors. She is well known for her ability to convey the essence of the wisdom teachings of yoga with exceptional clarity, insight, and relevance to students of all levels and from all walks of life. Teaching for close to two decades, Barrie shares the depth of her experience and knowledge to reveal a uniquely accessible, authentic, and integrated approach to yoga. She empowers students with tools to deepen their understanding and inspires them to embrace asana as a path for expansive self-discovery and inner growth.

Barrie is the creator of *The Skillful Yogi*, a thriving online practice and study community of yoga students and teachers with members from nine countries on four continents. Her book, *Evolving Your Yoga: Ten Principles for Enlightened Practice,* with foreword by Sophie Gregoire Trudeau, is a guide for teachers and continuing students to deepen, expand, and integrate the benefits of yoga in their lives.

A seasoned trainer and mentor of new teachers, Barrie serves on several teacher-training faculties in Canada and the

US. She is the creator of professional development courses, retreats, and mentoring programs for yoga teachers.

From 2011-2016, Barrie was the cofounder and codirector of Shri Yoga, Montreal's seminal place for the practice of alignment-based, heart-centered Hatha Yoga. A certified Anusara Yoga teacher, from 2003-2012 she was a Senior Anusara Yoga teacher and teacher-trainer. From 2006-2012, Barrie led Anusara Yoga events throughout Canada, the US, and internationally and served on the Anusara Yoga Teacher Certification Committee, mentoring new teachers toward certification.

Barrie is the co-creator of the *World Spine Care Yoga Project*, whose mission is to bring the benefits of posture, breathing, and mindfulness as a tool for pain management and active selfcare to low-mobility populations around the world. For more information, visit www.barrierisman.com, www. evolvingyouryoga.com, and the World Spine Care Yoga Project.

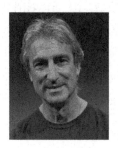

Richard Rosen began his study of yoga in 1980 and started teaching full time in 1987. He's a graduate of the B.K.S Iyengar Yoga Institute in San Francisco. For more than twenty years, he was a Contributing Editor with *Yoga Journal* magazine, for which he wrote feature articles, book and DVD reviews, and short columns. He's also the author of five books on yoga, the latest titled *Yoga FAQ: Almost Everything You Need to Know about Yoga—from Asanas to Yamas* (Shambhala, 2017). Richard lives in Berkeley, California. His website is: https://www.richardrosenyoga.com

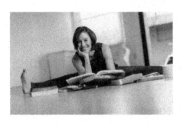 **Rachel Scott** is a teacher-trainer and author with more than 4,500 hours under her belt. Rachel is committed to helping her students uncover and express their voice, passion, and potential. After directing the Teachers College for a national yoga company for more than seven years (YYoga), Rachel left her corporate position to pursue a new mission—helping yoga teachers and studios around the world thrive in their businesses by elevating the quality and potency of their education offerings. She leverages her extensive academic training (MSci Instructional Systems and Learning Technologies, BA Columbia University) with more than two decades of yoga practice and business experience to help yoga studios and teachers reach their potential. She is a business thought partner and ally and brings more than fifteen years of experience as a teacher, teacher manager, studio director, program developer, and departmental director to the table. In addition to offering one-on-one coaching and mentoring, she offers several products to help trainers get their programs off the ground.

As a trainer, she is feisty, fun, inspirational, and knowledgeable. With keen insight into yoga training, she has a knack for helping yogis build the pragmatic skills they need to share their own teaching voice with confidence. She has contributed to *Yoga International*, the *Huffington Post*, and *Half Moon* and has taught at the *Omega Institute*, *Wanderlust*, the *Victoria Yoga Conference*, and more. Her books include *Wit and Wisdom From the Yoga Mat* (2017), *Head Over Heels: A Yogi's Guide to Dating* (2018), *Speedy Yoga* (2019), *Small Book of Yoga Practices* (2020), and *Yoga To Stay Young* (2020).

Visit her free resource library for teachers on YouTube at rachelscottyoga. Find out more and explore her extensive teaching, business, and training blog at http://www.rachelyoga.com.

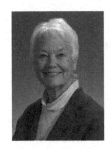

Dr. Anne Shumway-Cook, PT, PhD, FAPTA is a Professor Emeritus in the Department of Rehabilitation Medicine at the University of Washington, Seattle, Washington. Her research focused on understanding the physiologic basis for balance and mobility disorders in neurologic and geriatric populations and the translation of this research into best clinical practices for assessing and treating balance to reduce falls and optimize mobility function. She has developed a number of hospital and community evidence-based fall prevention programs. She has published extensively, and, along with Dr. Marjorie Woollacott, coauthored the textbook *Motor Control: Translating Research into Clinical Practice*. She has practiced meditation for more than forty-five years.

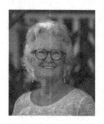

Priscilla Shumway, M.Ed was an award winning corporate trainer for over 25 years. Traveling nationally and internationally she conducted programs on Train the Trainer, Presentation Skills, Instructional Design, Facilitation Skills and several other custom programs. She has been a contributing author in 5 books on education and training. She was the co-editor with Kathy Hurley on <u>Real Women, Real Leaders</u> published by Wiley Publishing. A yoga student for over 18 years she is thrilled to be working collaboratively with these authors to write *Embrace Your Wobbles*.

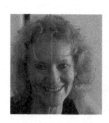

Jo Ann Staugaard-Jones, author and international movement educator, is a Full Professor of Kinesiology and Dance, an advanced Pilates teacher, an ERYT 500 Hatha Yoga Instructor (Shambhava School of Yoga, Colorado & the Himalayan Institute), a Yoga Anatomy instructor, and a teacher -trainer. Her degrees in Dance (NYU) and Movement Education (Kansas University) and experiences as a professional dancer and choreographer eventually led her to authorship of the *Anatomy of Exercise*

& Movement and the *Vital Psoas Muscle* by Lotus Publishing and North Atlantic Books. Her latest book, the *Concise Book of Yoga Anatomy,* was released in the fall of 2015.

Jo Ann has taught throughout the US, the UK, Sweden, the Netherlands, Prague, Costa Rica, and France. Believing knowledge of the body is a pathway to health and healing is her main focus in all her teachings. She is a member of Yoga Alliance, the International Yoga Therapy Association, the International Association of Dance Medicine & Science, and the Performing Arts Medicine Association (PAMA), where she has taught numerous workshops at worldwide conferences. She also sponsors holistic retreats and developed www.move-live.com, an interactive website to help inspire people to *keep moving*!

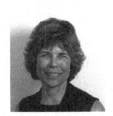

Dr. Marjorie Hines Woollacott, PhD, has been a neuroscience professor at the University of Oregon for more than three decades and a meditator for almost four. She also has a Master's degree in Asian Studies. Her research has been funded by the National Institutes of Health and the National Science Foundation and includes research in posture and balance control and testing the efficacy of alternative forms of therapy such as tai chi and meditation for improving attention and balance in adults. Along with Dr. Anne Shumway-Cook, she coauthored a popular textbook for health professionals and has written more than 180 peer-reviewed research articles, several of which were on meditation, the topic that motivated her to write her latest book, *Infinite Awareness: The Awakening of a Scientific Mind*. She was the keynote speaker at conferences in North and South America, Europe, Australia, and Asia and has taught courses not only in neuroscience and rehabilitation medicine, but in meditation, hatha yoga, and alternative and complementary medicine.

Her website is: https://marjoriewoollacott.com

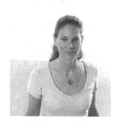 **Christine Wushke** has spent more than twenty years helping people find wellness and spiritual transformation. She specializes in Myofascial Massage, Myofascial Yoga, Reiki, and spiritual coaching. Her book, *Freedom is Your Nature*, was published by Inner Splendor Media in 2013. She runs *Journey to Light Wellness*, located in Okotoks AB, which offers myofascial yoga classes, meditation classes, transformational workshops, myofascial massage sessions, and hakomi therapy. For more information, visit http://freelyhuman.com/ okotoks-yoga-class-schedule/ and https://freelyhuman.com/ blog/.

References

CHAPTER 1: ALWAYS A BEGINNER

Fitts PM, Posner MI. Human performance. Belmont, CA: Brooks/Cole, 1967.

Exploring the therapeutic effects of yoga and its ability to increase quality of life: International Journal of Yoga 2011.

Catherine Woodyard

Yoga: What You Need to Know: National Center for Complimentary and integrative Health 2018

CHAPTER 2: WHY WOBBLES MATTER

1. This network includes areas of the medial prefrontal cortex, the posterior cingulate cortex, the precuneus, the inferior parietal lobe, and the lateral temporal cortex.

2. This network includes the anterior insula and the anterior cingulate cortex. It regulates subjectively perceived feelings, which might, for instance, lead to being distracted during

a task. The salience network is thought to play a vital role in detecting novel events and in switching activity during meditation among assemblies of neurons that make up the brain's large-scale networks. It may shift attention away from the default-mode network, for instance.

3. The dorsolateral prefrontal cortex, which is part of the executive attention network (contributing to working memory and management of cognitive processes), and the lateral inferior parietal lobe, used in interpreting sensory information.

4. The dorsolateral prefrontal cortex, which contributes to executive attention.

5. The prefrontal cortex modulates or inhibits our limbic system, our emotional system (which means that if we have a weak prefrontal cortex, we are emotionally reactive). In challenging situations, our ability to recover equanimity (or resilience) is reduced. It is the attentional networks of the prefrontal cortex that are strengthened by meditation, thus making us less reactive to emotional stresses.

6. Neural circuitry of compassion includes activity in the dorsolateral prefrontal cortex and increased activity in the anterior cingulate cortex, associated with positive feelings and decreased activity in the amygdala, which is associated with distress.

Ricard M., Lutz A., Davidson, RJ. <u>Mind of the meditator.</u> *Scientific American*, 2014 Nov; 311(5):38-45.

Shumway-Cook A, Woollacott M., *Motor Control: Translating Research into Clinical Practice*, 5th Edition. Baltimore: Wolters Kluwer, 2016.

CHAPTER 8: BALANCE, MEMORY AND EAGLE POSE

Zettel-Watson

https://www.ncbi.nlm.nih.gov/pubmed/26694752

bioRxiv

Buschman, et al., 2011; Cowan, 2010; Luck and Vogel, 1997; Ma et al., 2014

Acknowledgements

To Dr. Anne Shumway-Cook, my sister and reviewer. From an early age she taught me the difference between a nickel and a dime (Did you know the nickel is worth more because it is bigger?) and so many more valuable lessons in life. Our weekly calls have delved into so many issues; from raising boys and grandchildren, to unconditional love (even during those moments when you don't feel it), to spiritual practices. This book would not have existed without her great skill at rewriting my stream of consciousness and putting it into words that connect. Her continual encouragement spurred me on when life's wobbles often got in the way of finishing the book.

Her textbook and research partner and friend Marjorie Woollacott was also instrumental in crafting edits to a number of these essays. Marjorie's daily yoga and meditation practice and her research into the science behind it laid much of the groundwork for this book.

To my yoga teachers, wherever you are; whether I practiced with you for 15 years or for one amazing session while traveling out of town. Each of you has added to my love of this practice. Each of you has added a new dimension, a new nugget for thought. My current yoga sangha, Holy Cow Yoga in Charleston, SC is a spiritual home that commits to going beyond the physical practice and supporting the full 8 limbs of yogic philosophy. Their commitment to "making this your own practice" is not often found in studios where hot yoga and power yoga are the norm.

To my "3 boys", my two sons and my loving husband of over 40 years. Your unconditional love and support are what sustains me. Watching your lives unfold with grace, humor and love for your families lets me know I have done my job. You have been an essential part of my spiritual path and my yoga practice and you continue to deepen it for me. I hope that the wisdom from my yoga mat has and will continue to guide my path forward.

Illustrations: Maryori Hernandez through Upwork.com

Made in USA - Kendallville, IN
1200758_9781647042509
11.28.2020 0850